Current Challenges and Personalized Treatment in Cardiovascular Disease

Current Challenges and Personalized Treatment in Cardiovascular Disease

Editor

Georgios Samanidis

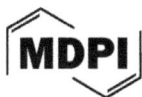

Basel • Beijing • Wuhan • Barcelona • Belgrade • Novi Sad • Cluj • Manchester

Editor
Georgios Samanidis
Onassis Cardiac Surgery
Center
Athens
Greece

Editorial Office
MDPI AG
Grosspeteranlage 5
4052 Basel, Switzerland

This is a reprint of articles from the Special Issue published online in the open access journal *Journal of Clinical Medicine* (ISSN 2077-0383) (available at: https://www.mdpi.com/journal/jpm/special_issues/Challenges_Cardiovascular).

For citation purposes, cite each article independently as indicated on the article page online and as indicated below:

Lastname, A.A.; Lastname, B.B. Article Title. *Journal Name* **Year**, *Volume Number*, Page Range.

ISBN 978-3-7258-1889-1 (Hbk)
ISBN 978-3-7258-1890-7 (PDF)
doi.org/10.3390/books978-3-7258-1890-7

© 2024 by the authors. Articles in this book are Open Access and distributed under the Creative Commons Attribution (CC BY) license. The book as a whole is distributed by MDPI under the terms and conditions of the Creative Commons Attribution-NonCommercial-NoDerivs (CC BY-NC-ND) license.

Contents

About the Editor vii

Preface ix

George Samanidis
Current Challenges in Diagnosis and Treatment of Cardiovascular Disease
Reprinted from: *J. Pers. Med.* **2024**, *14*, 786, doi:10.3390/jpm14080786 1

George Samanidis, Meletios Kanakis and Konstantinos Perreas
Outcomes after Transcatheter Mitral Valve Implantation: A Literature Review
Reprinted from: *J. Pers. Med.* **2022**, *12*, 2074, doi:10.3390/jpm12122074 5

Justyna Chojdak-Łukasiewicz, Sławomir Budrewicz and Marta Waliszewska-Prosół
Cerebral Aneurysms Caused by Atrial Myxoma—A Systematic Review of the Literature
Reprinted from: *J. Pers. Med.* **2023**, *13*, 8, doi:10.3390/jpm13010008 15

Tiziano Torre, Alberto Pozzoli, Marco Valgimigli, Laura Anna Leo, Francesca Toto, Mirko Muretti, et al.
Minimally Invasive Isolated and Hybrid Surgical Revascularization for Multivessel Coronary Disease: A Single-Center Long-Term Follow-Up
Reprinted from: *J. Pers. Med.* **2024**, *14*, 528, doi:10.3390/jpm14050528 29

Paraskevi Zotou, Aris Bechlioulis, Spyridon Tsiouris, Katerina K. Naka, Xanthi Xourgia, Konstantinos Pappas, et al.
The Role of Myocardial Perfusion Imaging in the Prediction of Major Adverse Cardiovascular Events at 1 Year Follow-Up: A Single Center's Experience
Reprinted from: *J. Pers. Med.* **2023**, *13*, 871, doi:10.3390/jpm13050871 42

Eleni Spiropoulou, George Samanidis, Meletios Kanakis and Ioannis Nenekidis
Risk Factors for Acute Postoperative Delirium in Cardiac Surgery Patients >65 Years Old
Reprinted from: *J. Pers. Med.* **2022**, *12*, 1529, doi:10.3390/jpm12091529 51

Sebastian D. Sahli, Alexander Kaserer, Julia Braun, Raed Aser, Donat R. Spahn and Markus J. Wilhelm
A Descriptive Analysis of Hybrid Cannulated Extracorporeal Life Support
Reprinted from: *J. Pers. Med.* **2024**, *14*, 179, doi:10.3390/jpm14020179 60

Emyal Alyaydin, Juergen Reinhard Sindermann, Jeanette Köppe, Joachim Gerss, Patrik Dröge, Thomas Ruhnke, et al.
Depression and Anxiety in Heart Transplant Recipients: Prevalence and Impact on Post-Transplant Outcomes
Reprinted from: *J. Pers. Med.* **2023**, *13*, 844, doi:10.3390/jpm13050844 72

Yoonkyung Chang, Min Kyoung Kang, Moo-Seok Park, Gwang-Hyun Leem and Tae-Jin Song
Resolved Proteinuria May Attenuate the Risk of Heart Failure: A Nationwide Population-Based Cohort Study
Reprinted from: *J. Pers. Med.* **2023**, *13*, 1662, doi:10.3390/jpm13121662 83

Akira Sezai, Hisakuni Sekino, Makoto Taoka, Shunji Osaka and Masashi Tanaka
A Comparative Study to Investigate the Effects of Bisoprolol in Patients with Chronic Heart Failure and Hypertension When Switched from Tablets to Transdermal Patches
Reprinted from: *J. Pers. Med.* **2023**, *13*, 785, doi:10.3390/jpm13050785 92

Bárbara Luque, Naima Z. Farhane-Medina, Marta Villalba, Rosario Castillo-Mayén, Esther Cuadrado and Carmen Tabernero
Positivity and Health Locus of Control: Key Variables to Intervene on Well-Being of Cardiovascular Disease Patients
Reprinted from: *J. Pers. Med.* **2023**, *13*, 873, doi:10.3390/jpm13050873 . . . . **101**

Chung-Hsin Yeh, Fung-Chang Sung, Chih-Hsin Muo, Pao-Sheng Yen and Chung Y. Hsu
Stroke Risk in Young Women with Primary Dysmenorrhea: A Propensity-Score-Matched Retrospective Cohort Study
Reprinted from: *J. Pers. Med.* **2023**, *13*, 114, doi:10.3390/jpm13010114 . . . . **116**

About the Editor

Georgios Samanidis

    I graduated from the Medical School of the University of Athens, completed my training in Cardiothoracic Surgery in Greece, and was awarded a PhD at the Medical School of the University of Athens, Greece. I have been working at the Onassis Cardiac Surgery Center in Athens, Greece, in the Department of Cardiac Surgery for 17 years. I have performed many cardiac surgery operations as a consultant. My interests are aortic surgery, heart valve disease, minimally invasive cardiac surgery, and biomarkers in heart disease. My special interests are minimally invasive thoracoscopic cardiac surgery, original research, and evidence-based medicine.

Preface

Innovative diagnostic and therapeutic approaches for patients with heart disease are available. Artificial intelligence is introducing a new era of clinical research. Artificial intelligence cannot replace the original data collection process alone; however, it can support other stages of data analysis and paper presentation. At present, many articles are published with the support of artificial intelligence. Authors, reviewers, and editors should review every scientific presentation submitted and read in any forum or journal.

Acknowledgments: The Guest Editor would like to express their thanks to the Assistant Editor Mrs Emmy Yu for her support in preparing this Special Issue. Moreover, thanks are given to all authors for their contribution of updated and intriguing articles to this Special Issue.

Georgios Samanidis
Editor

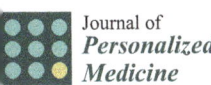

Editorial

Current Challenges in Diagnosis and Treatment of Cardiovascular Disease

George Samanidis

Department of Adult Cardiac Surgery, Onassis Cardiac Surgery Center, 17674 Athens, Greece; gsamanidis@yahoo.gr; Tel.: +30-2109493832

Citation: Samanidis, G. Current Challenges in Diagnosis and Treatment of Cardiovascular Disease. *J. Pers. Med.* **2024**, *14*, 786. https://doi.org/10.3390/jpm14080786

Received: 7 July 2024
Accepted: 23 July 2024
Published: 25 July 2024

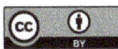

Copyright: © 2024 by the author. Licensee MDPI, Basel, Switzerland. This article is an open access article distributed under the terms and conditions of the Creative Commons Attribution (CC BY) license (https://creativecommons.org/licenses/by/4.0/).

Cardiovascular disease is a leading the cause of death worldwide among the various cardiac pathologies that directly or indirectly affect the quality of life of patients. A current challenge in the management of cardiovascular disease is combining known clinical practice with updated diagnostic methods and treatment. Artificial intelligence may offer an alternative diagnostic approach for treating patients with cardiac disease, but alone and without clinician support, it may have limited application.

Cardiovascular disease is a leading cause of death worldwide [1]. A wide spectrum of cardiac pathologies directly or indirectly affect the quality of life of patients. Coronary artery disease, heart valve disease, thoracic aorta disease, heart rhythm disease and cardio-oncology are the most common heart pathologies. The diagnostic approaches used for treating these syndromes have changed in the last few years. Noninvasive diagnostics methods for heart disease diagnosis, such as coronary artery computed tomography (CT), cardiac CT, cardiac magnetic resonance imaging (MRI) and cardiac positron emission tomography (PET), are prominent strategies present in the armentaria of cardiologists, radiologists and cardiac surgeons [2–4]. Moreover, less invasive intervention techniques [transcather aortic valve implantation (TAVI), transcather mitral valve implantation (TMVI), Mitral-clip, endovascular thoracic and aortic arch branched stenting] allow patients to receive the most up-to-date treatment with acceptable short-, mid- and long-term results [5–8]. Unlike in the past, nowadays, inoperable patients or patients with a high or prohibitive perioperative cardiac surgery risk can be treated with modern transcather techniques. Improving the quality of mechanical circulatory support devices contributes to improved quality of life in patients with acute or chronic heart failure [9,10]. The number of patients with congenital heart disease who previously underwent heart surgery and adult patients with congenital heart disease will increase in the next few years. An accurate diagnostic approach in patients with acquired and congenital heart disease will be needed to ensure the best medical or intervention treatment. Also, the prevention of coronary artery disease and identification of patients with silent ischemic heart disease may reduce the number of patients admitted in hospital with acute symptoms and avoid ischemic heart complications. In future, older patients will constitute the majority of patients with heart disease in need of cardiology or cardiac surgery interventions. The comorbidities of these patients will be crucial point for treatment. Postoperative psychological dysfunction is identified as a risk factor for worse outcomes in patients who underwent major cardiac surgery in [11]. The early identification and treatment of these patients may improve perioperative and long-term results.

Nowadays, the primary treatment approaches used in interventional cardiology and cardiac surgery are transcather intervention in heart valve disease and either minimally invasive cardiac surgery or a hybrid approach in coronary artery disease and structural heart disease (aortic, mitral and tricuspid valves) [5,12,13]. Although transcatheter aortic valve implantation (TAVI) was introduced over 15 years ago, its long-term results regarding quality of life are still debated through comparison to the results of surgical aortic valve replacement. On the other hand, patients facing high or prohibitive risk in open cardiac surgery are suitable for TAVI with acceptable mid-term results. Severe mitral valve regurgitation in patients at high risk during an operation requires them to have alternative options for treatment by transcather mitral valve implantation (TMVI) [14]. Moreover, patients with severe mitral valve annulus calcification (MAC) who are not candidates for operation constitute a population suitable for TMVI. Many prosthetic mitral valves for TMVI have been developed. The short-term results after TMVI are encouraging, but the mid- and long-term results are unknown.

Minimizing surgical stress enables the fast recovery of patients who underwent major heart surgery [15]. Minimal invasive cardiac surgery (MICS) for aortic and mitral correction or replacement by a thoracoscopic approach are alternative surgical approaches. Making a small skin incision and avoiding median sternotomy reduces surgical stress and contributes to the early mobilization of patients after operation. These advantages prevent early postoperative complications such as lung atelectasis and pneumonia. Furthermore, an MICS approach reduces postoperative pain, which improves pulmonary function postoperatively. Short-, mid- and long-term results are similar with an open-sternum approach.

Coronary artery bypass grafting (CABG) remains the most common cardiac surgery procedure. On the other hand, a hybrid approach for treating severe coronary artery disease may offer better long-term results compared with percutaneous coronary intervention or optimal medical treatment in selective patients with coronary artery disease. Although the number of patients treated with a hybrid revascularization approach worldwide is small, the outcomes in these patients are promising [12]. More studies are needed to confirm these results and enable this method's acceptance as a revascularization strategy in patients with severe coronary artery disease.

Diagnostic approaches used for the treatment of patients with progressive heart failure (HF) face many challenges [16–18]. Patients with preserved or non-preserved heart failure constitute large populations who need special therapy approaches. The use of alternative drug administration to achieve the optimum drug affect is well described by Sezai et al. [16]. Although the number of patients in this study is small and it has many weaknesses, the use of a transdermal patch for drug administration may be more effective than oral administration in patients with arterial hypertension and heart failure. Limited data are available about mental disorders and outcomes in patients undergoing heart transplantation or supported by mechanical circulatory support. Alyaydin et al., in their study, present the incidence of depression and anxiety in heart transplant patients [17]. The authors conclude that these patients have worse outcomes compared with patients without mental disorders. The study shows that chronic diseases including chronic heart disease affect direct quality of life and outcomes. A priority for the prevention of heart disease is the identification of patients in the early stage of progressive of heart disease. Chang et al. show that proteinuria may be a possible predictor of heart failure [18].

The many innovative diagnostic and treatment approaches for heart disease could also lead to a new era in medicine and cardiovascular disease. The use of up-to-date prosthetic heart valve devices for the transcatheter treatment of heart valve disease improves patient outcomes. Minimally invasive cardiac surgery minimizes surgical stress, and its use is a growing trend in cardiac surgery. On the other hand, the use of artificial intelligence in diagnostic methods (such as CT, MRI and transthoracic and transesophageal echocardiography) and diagnostic algorithms for heart disease diagnosis in routine clinical practice is currently a hot topic in cardiology and cardiac surgery [19–23]. Using artificial intelligence for the early identification of patients with severe heart disease and prediction of outcomes in these patients may improve such outcomes. Although artificial intelligence is hot topic in current medical practice, the clinical examination of patients, identification of crucial symptoms in patients, selection of laboratory tests and appropriate diagnostic examination remain the most significant elements of good medical practice. The application of artificial intelligence may offer the best diagnostic approach for patients with severe heart disease.

An interesting review about the possible cause of cerebral aneurysm is presented by Chojdak-Łukasiewicz et al. [24]. The authors, in their study, list cases of patients with coexisting he cardiac myxoma and cerebral aneurysm. The proposed cause of cerebral aneurysm formation is cerebral artery embolism or vascular inflammation due interleukin secretion from cardiac myxoma. No guidelines exist regarding the management and treatment of these patients. On the other hand, complete surgical excision remains the treatment of choice of patients with cardiac myxoma.

Yeh et al. compare woman of reproductive age with and without primary dysmenorrhea [25]. The authors present a large study population in comparative groups. In this study, the authors evaluate primary dysmenorrhea as a possible risk factor for late stroke. They conclude that dysmenorrhea is risk factor for stroke (ischemic and hemorrhagic) and affects patients' quality of life.

In conclusion, the main challenge in the management of cardiovascular disease is the combination of known clinical practice with up-to-date diagnostic methods and treatments. Artificial intelligence may offer an alternative diagnostic approach for treating patients with cardiac disease, but alone and without clinician support, it may have limited application.

Funding: This research received no external funding.

Conflicts of Interest: No conflicts of interests have been declared.

References

1. Zotou, P.; Bechlioulis, A.; Tsiouris, S.; Naka, K.K.; Xourgia, X.; Pappas, K.; Lakkas, L.; Rammos, A.; Kalef-Ezra, J.; Michalis, L.K.; et al. The Role of Myocardial Perfusion Imaging in the Prediction of Major Adverse Cardiovascular Events at 1 Year Follow-Up: A Single Center's Experience. *J. Pers. Med.* **2023**, *13*, 871. [CrossRef] [PubMed] [PubMed Central]
2. Schultz, J.; van den Hoogen, I.J.; Kuneman, J.H.; de Graaf, M.A.; Kamperidis, V.; Broersen, A.; Jukema, J.W.; Sakellarios, A.; Nikopoulos, S.; Tsarapatsani, K.; et al. Coronary computed tomography angiography-based endothelial wall shear stress in normal coronary arteries. *Int. J. Cardiovasc. Imaging* **2023**, *39*, 441–450. [CrossRef] [PubMed] [PubMed Central]
3. Sun, Z.; Silberstein, J.; Vaccarezza, M. Cardiovascular Computed Tomography in the Diagnosis of Cardiovascular Disease: Beyond Lumen Assessment. *J. Cardiovasc. Dev. Dis.* **2024**, *11*, 22. [CrossRef] [PubMed] [PubMed Central]
4. Nayfeh, M.; Ahmed, A.I.; Saad, J.M.; Alahdab, F.; Al-Mallah, M. The Role of Cardiac PET in Diagnosis and Prognosis of Ischemic Heart Disease: Optimal Modality Across Different Patient Populations. *Curr. Atheroscler. Rep.* **2023**, *25*, 351–357. [CrossRef] [PubMed] [PubMed Central]
5. Thyregod, H.G.H.; Jørgensen, T.H.; Ihlemann, N.; Steinbrüchel, D.A.; Nissen, H.; Kjeldsen, B.J.; Petursson, P.; De Backer, O.; Olsen, P.S.; Søndergaard, L. Transcatheter or surgical aortic valve implantation: 10-year outcomes of the NOTION trial. *Eur. Heart J.* **2024**, *45*, 1116–1124. [CrossRef] [PubMed] [PubMed Central]
6. Samanidis, G.; Kanakis, M.; Perreas, K. Outcomes after Transcatheter Mitral Valve Implantation: A Literature Review. *J. Pers. Med.* **2022**, *12*, 2074. [CrossRef] [PubMed] [PubMed Central]
7. Zancanaro, E.; Buzzatti, N.; Denti, P.; Guicciardi, N.A.; Melillo, E.; Monaco, F.; Agricola, E.; Ancona, F.; Alfieri, O.; De Bonis, M.; et al. Eligibility to COAPT trial in the daily practice: A real-world experience. *Catheter. Cardiovasc. Interv.* **2024**, *epub ahead of print*. [CrossRef] [PubMed]
8. Deniz, G.; Kasımzade, F.; Ozcınar, E.; Yazicioglu, L.; Eryılmaz, S. Long-term outcomes of TEVAR for thoracic aortic diseases: A retrospective single-center study. *J. Cardiothorac. Surg.* **2024**, *19*, 405. [CrossRef] [PubMed] [PubMed Central]
9. Yin, M.Y.; Maneta, E.; Kyriakopoulos, C.P.; Michaels, A.T.; Genovese, L.D.; Indaram, M.B.; Wever-Pinzon, O.; Singh, R.; Tseliou, E.; Taleb, I.; et al. Cardiac Reverse Remodeling Mediated by HeartMate 3 Left Ventricular Assist Device: Comparison to Older Generation Devices. *ASAIO J.* **2024**, *epub ahead of print*. [CrossRef] [PubMed]
10. Sahli, S.D.; Kaserer, A.; Braun, J.; Aser, R.; Spahn, D.R.; Wilhelm, M.J. A Descriptive Analysis of Hybrid Cannulated Extracorporeal Life Support. *J. Pers. Med.* **2024**, *14*, 179. [CrossRef] [PubMed] [PubMed Central]
11. Spiropoulou, E.; Samanidis, G.; Kanakis, M.; Nenekidis, I. Risk Factors for Acute Postoperative Delirium in Cardiac Surgery Patients >65 Years Old. *J. Pers. Med.* **2022**, *12*, 1529. [CrossRef] [PubMed] [PubMed Central]
12. Torre, T.; Pozzoli, A.; Valgimigli, M.; Leo, L.A.; Toto, F.; Muretti, M.; Birova, S.; Ferrari, E.; Pedrazzini, G.; Demertzis, S. Minimally Invasive Isolated and Hybrid Surgical Revascularization for Multivessel Coronary Disease: A Single-Center Long-Term Follow-Up. *J. Pers. Med.* **2024**, *14*, 528. [CrossRef] [PubMed] [PubMed Central]
13. Farid, S.; Ali, J.M.; Stohlner, V.; Alam, R.; Schofield, P.; Nashef, S.; De Silva, R. Long-Term Outcome of Patients Undergoing Minimally Invasive Direct Coronary Artery Bypass Surgery: A Single-Center Experience. *Innovations* **2018**, *13*, 23–28. [CrossRef] [PubMed]
14. Farouk, H.; Schöne, D.; Witt, C.; Bayyud, H.; Kandil, M.; Kloppe, A. Papillary muscle rupture after transcatheter aortic valve implantation: A case report and literature review. *Catheter. Cardiovasc. Interv.* **2023**, *102*, 542–546. [CrossRef] [PubMed]

15. Lucà, F.; van Garsse, L.; Rao, C.M.; Parise, O.; La Meir, M.; Puntrello, C.; Rubino, G.; Carella, R.; Lorusso, R.; Gensini, G.F.; et al. Minimally invasive mitral valve surgery: A systematic review. *Minim. Invasive Surg.* **2013**, *2013*, 179569. [CrossRef] [PubMed] [PubMed Central]
16. Sezai, A.; Sekino, H.; Taoka, M.; Osaka, S.; Tanaka, M. A Comparative Study to Investigate the Effects of Bisoprolol in Patients with Chronic Heart Failure and Hypertension When Switched from Tablets to Transdermal Patches. *J. Pers. Med.* **2023**, *13*, 785. [CrossRef] [PubMed] [PubMed Central]
17. Alyaydin, E.; Sindermann, J.R.; Köppe, J.; Gerss, J.; Dröge, P.; Ruhnke, T.; Günster, C.; Reinecke, H.; Feld, J. Depression and Anxiety in Heart Transplant Recipients: Prevalence and Impact on Post-Transplant Outcomes. *J. Pers. Med.* **2023**, *13*, 844. [CrossRef] [PubMed] [PubMed Central]
18. Chang, Y.; Kang, M.K.; Park, M.S.; Leem, G.H.; Song, T.J. Resolved Proteinuria May Attenuate the Risk of Heart Failure: A Nationwide Population-Based Cohort Study. *J. Pers. Med.* **2023**, *13*, 1662. [CrossRef] [PubMed] [PubMed Central]
19. Kagiyama, N.; Abe, Y.; Kusunose, K.; Kato, N.; Kaneko, T.; Murata, A.; Ota, M.; Shibayama, K.; Izumo, M.; Watanabe, H. Multicenter validation study for automated left ventricular ejection fraction assessment using a handheld ultrasound with artificial intelligence. *Sci. Rep.* **2024**, *14*, 15359. [CrossRef] [PubMed] [PubMed Central]
20. Jafari, R.; Verma, R.; Aggarwal, V.; Gupta, R.K.; Singh, A. Deep learning-based segmentation of left ventricular myocardium on dynamic contrast-enhanced MRI: A comprehensive evaluation across temporal frames. *Int. J. Comput. Assist. Radiol. Surg.* **2024**, *epub ahead of print*. [CrossRef] [PubMed]
21. Sirset-Becker, T.; Clark, A.; Flaherty, J.D.; Mehta, C.K.; Allen, B.D.; McCarthy, P.M.; Pham, D.T.; Churyla, A.; Dasi, L.P.; Malaisrie, S.C. Modeling of Valve-in-Valve Transcatheter Aortic Valve Implantation after Aortic Root Replacement Using 3-Dimensional Artificial Intelligence Algorithm. *J. Thorac. Cardiovasc. Surg.* **2024**, *epub ahead of print*. [CrossRef] [PubMed]
22. Ahluwalia, M.; Kpodonu, J.; Agu, E. Risk Stratification in Hypertrophic Cardiomyopathy: Leveraging Artificial Intelligence to Provide Guidance in the Future. *JACC Adv.* **2023**, *2*, 100562. [CrossRef] [PubMed] [PubMed Central]
23. Akerman, A.P.; Porumb, M.; Scott, C.G.; Beqiri, A.; Chartsias, A.; Ryu, A.J.; Hawkes, W.; Huntley, G.D.; Arystan, A.Z.; Kane, G.C.; et al. Automated Echocardiographic Detection of Heart Failure with Preserved Ejection Fraction Using Artificial Intelligence. *JACC Adv.* **2023**, *2*, 100452. [CrossRef] [PubMed] [PubMed Central]
24. Chojdak-Łukasiewicz, J.; Budrewicz, S.; Waliszewska-Prosół, M. Cerebral Aneurysms Caused by Atrial Myxoma-A Systematic Review of the Literature. *J. Pers. Med.* **2022**, *13*, 8. [CrossRef] [PubMed] [PubMed Central]
25. Yeh, C.H.; Sung, F.C.; Muo, C.H.; Yen, P.S.; Hsu, C.Y. Stroke Risk in Young Women with Primary Dysmenorrhea: A Propensity-Score-Matched Retrospective Cohort Study. *J. Pers. Med.* **2023**, *13*, 114. [CrossRef] [PubMed] [PubMed Central]

Disclaimer/Publisher's Note: The statements, opinions and data contained in all publications are solely those of the individual author(s) and contributor(s) and not of MDPI and/or the editor(s). MDPI and/or the editor(s) disclaim responsibility for any injury to people or property resulting from any ideas, methods, instructions or products referred to in the content.

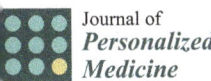

Review

Outcomes after Transcatheter Mitral Valve Implantation: A Literature Review

George Samanidis [1,*], Meletios Kanakis [2] and Konstantinos Perreas [1]

1. Department of Adult Cardiac Surgery, Onassis Cardiac Surgery Center, 356 Leoforos Syggrou, 17674 Athens, Greece
2. Department of Pediatric and Congenital Heart Surgery, Onassis Cardiac Surgery Center, 356 Leoforos Syggrou, 17674 Athens, Greece
* Correspondence: gsamanidis@yahoo.gr; Tel.: +30-0032109493832

Abstract: Mitral valve disease is the most common heart valve disease worldwide. Surgical mitral valve replacement or repair has been an established therapy in patients with severe mitral valve disease for many years. On the other hand, many patients with advanced mitral valve disease and severe comorbidities are treated conservatively and are excluded from the surgical procedure. Furthermore, in patients with severe comorbidities, transcatheter mitral valve repair by edge-to-edge technique with MitraClip or transcatheter mitral valve repair with a non-absorbable ring have been added as therapeutic options over the last few years. Alternative procedures for the treatment of patients with advanced prosthetic or native mitral valve diseases include transcatheter access for replacement or implantation of a new prosthetic valve in the diseased mitral valve. Promising results were published about short-term outcomes of patients who underwent the transcatheter mitral valve replacement. The current view and results of the transcatheter mitral valve implantation in patients with advanced native or prosthetic mitral valve disease are briefly discussed.

Keywords: transcatheter; mitral valve; replacement; implantation

1. Introduction

Mitral valve disease (MVD) is the most common heart valve disease (HVD) worldwide [1–3]. In developed countries, the dominant MVD are primary and secondary mitral regurgitation, while in developing and other countries it is rheumatic disease. In patients with untreated mitral valve pathology, the progressive worsening of left ventricular dysfunction and development of fixed pulmonary hypertension affect morbidity and mortality [1–3]. Surgery remains the treatment of choice for symptomatic mitral valve regurgitation (MR), mitral stenosis (MS) and mixed mitral valve disease (MMVD) [1–3]. Surgical mitral valve replacement (sMVR) in patients with MS or MMVD has been an established technique for many years, while surgical mitral valve repair (MVr) is suggested as the gold standard operative technique for patients with MR [1,2]. Many patients with advanced MVD and severe comorbidities such as previous cardiac surgery are treated conservatively and are excluded from the surgical procedure. This conservative approach may affect the survival rate of these patients. An alternative procedure for MVD treatment has been proposed and includes the transcatheter access of the mitral valve for repair or implantation of theprosthetic valve device in the diseased mitral valve (MV) [4–7]. Patients directed to MVr by edge-to-edge technique with mitraclip or transcatheter MVr with a non-absorbable ring constitute the largest population for these aforementioned techniques and patients directed to transcatheter mitral valve implantation (TMVI) represent the minority [7–10]. Nowadays, controversial results have been reported about short- and mid-term results of patients who underwent the TMVI [8–10]. Moreover, the off label indication for TMVI is the degeneration of the bio-prosthetic mitral valve. Degenerated bio-prosthetic mitral valves will be another challenge for the therapeutic approach in the future due to the increasing number of patients who underwent sMVR in the past [9,11,12]. First TMVI was reported in 2012 with CardiAQ valve (Edwards Life Sciences, Irvine, California, United States) [13]. Nowadays, a significant number of new mitral devices are tested for durability and effectiveness during follow-up.

2. Methods

This review evaluates the current challenges of transcatheter mitral valve replacement or implantation in patients with advanced mitral valve disease. PubMed was used for searching publications regarding the outcomes of patients after TMVI. The chronic period for data extraction was 2013–2022. This review includes studies with reported outcomes after TMVI. "Transcatheter mitral valve implantation" or "transcatheter mitral valve replacement" and "outcomes" were used as key words for searching on the PubMed site. The perioperative morbidity and mortality reports after TMVI were outcomes of interest. However, the TMVI procedure is a relevant new technique for mitral valve disease treatment and minimal data are available for safe analysis.

3. Results

3.1. Indication for Transcatheter Mitral Valve Implantation

The most common indication for TMVI is advanced MVD due to severe secondary MR with reduced left ventricle ejection fraction (LVEF) and heart failure (HF), severe mitral annulus or mitral leaflet calcification, severe mixed mitral valve pathology with small mitral valve orifice area, degenerated bio-prosthetic mitral valve disease and failed MVr (ring annuloplasty) [14,15]. In addition, patients with severe comorbidities and high operative risk are considered as candidates for TMVI [14,15]. Patients with symptomatic primary MR and asymptomatic MR with left ventricle (LV) dysfunction are the ideal candidates for surgical MVr, while patients with secondary moderate to severe and symptomatic MR are candidates for various treatment modalities such as medical treatment alone, transcatheter repair (edge-to edge technique, repair), and transcatheter repair with medical treatment to SMVR [1–3]. The recent studies demonstrated that outcomes (hospitalization and mortality rate during 1 and 2 years of follow-up) of patients with secondary MR who were treated by transcatheter MVr and medical treatment did not differ compared to the medical treatment only [16,17]. On the other hand, Stone et al. reported that the transcatheter MVr had a lower rate for hospitalization and all-cause mortality within 2 years versus the medical treatment alone [18].

3.2. Methods for Transcatheter Mitral Valve Implantation

Two methods for the catheter-based mitral valve implantation have been proposed over the last few years, and these are the transapical and transfemoral/transseptal approach [13,15]. In both techniques, the prosthetic valve is implanted in the native or prosthetic pathological mitral valve under guidance of the transesophageal echocardiography (TEE), ideally in a hybrid room. Transfemoral access is considered a less invasive technique due to lower peri-procedural complications and mortality rates than the transapical access [19,20]. The transfemoral access is achieved by puncturing the common femoral vein under guidance of ultrasonography and finally the insertion of the large diameter sheath for the delivering system of the prosthetic mitral valve [15,16,20]. On the other hand, the transapical implantation needs a small left anterior thoracotomy and small incision in the LV for inserting the delivery system of prosthetic valve through the LV apex with the subsequent implantation of the prosthetic valve in the mitral annulus [21]. The most common prosthetic mitral valves, which have been reported for TMVI are the CardiAQ-Edwards TMVR System (Edwards Lifesciences, Irvine, CA, USA), EVOQUE TMVR System (Edwards Lifesciences, Irvine, CA, USA), SAPIEN M3 System (Edwards Lifesciences, Irvine, CA, USA), Cardiovalve TMVR system (Cardiovalve Ltd., Or Yehuda, Israel), Tiara TMVR System (Neovasc Inc., Richmond, BC, Canada), Tendyne Mitral Valve System (Abbott Vascular, Roseville, MN, USA), INTREPID TMVR System (Medtronic,

Inc., Redwood City, CA, USA), Caisson TMVR system (LivaNova PLC, London, UK), and HighLife TMVR system (HighLife Medical, Paris, France) [21–23]. The early results after TMVI demonstrated the promising short-term results regarding early morbidity and 30-day mortality, while the mid- and long-term results after implantation are expected in the next 3–5 years [19–23]. Long-term durability of devices, left ventricle outflow tract (LVOT) obstruction during or after procedure, and early and late prosthetic valve thrombosis after implantation are the most common difficulties and complications that should be solved by manufacturers, researchers, and clinicians [14,20–23]. New prosthetic valves and delivered devices for TMVI have been developed by many institutions and manufacturers worldwide with promising results [23]. At this time, advantages and disadvantages of the prosthetic valve, which is used in TMVI, is difficult to present due to the limited implanted prosthetic valves and limited number of patients who treated with these techniques. About other valves, minimal data are available about the routine practice for using these valves, due to the limited number of valves that were implanted. Some results after the TMVI implantation is available in patients who were received Sapien (balloon-expandable) and Tendyne (self-expanding) valves. On the other hand, these cannot be compared in practice because the implantation technique is different between the two valves. For implanting, the Tendyne valve needs a mini right thoracotomy and it is a different philosophy from the percutaneous valve implantation, which is used in the Sapien valve. Although Tendyne is included in TMVI, the delivery system of the Tendyne valve is inserted via a small incision in the left ventricle apex. In practice, it is a different approach from the percutaneous valve implantation. Furthermore, in the Sapien, the valve implantation is used knowing the delivery system such as in the TAVI, and it is for the off-label use for the prosthetic mitral valve degeneration pathology and in case with MVr failure or advanced mitral annulus calcification (MAC). Moreover, the second study with some short- and mid-term results was presented after the Intrepid valve implantation, and it regarded only 50 patients. Mid- and long-term outcomes of the current development clinical trial are expected to confirm the preliminary acceptable short-term results after TMVI, which have been announced in published materials in the past.

3.3. Outcomes of Patients after Transcatheter Mitral Valve Replacement or Implantation

Most of the patients that underwent TMVI have severe comorbidities, which affect the length of stay in hospitals and the ICU. In-hospital mortality and all-cause mortality are also increasing due to more advanced cardiac pathologies (coexisting heart failure, permanent atrial fibrillation, pulmonary artery hypertension and previous cardiac surgery). Transapical (TA) mitral valve implantation is the newest TMVI technique and is used in patients with a high risk for operation. The published results are encouraging regarding mortality and morbidity. On the other hand, most of these patients included in these studies were patients with severe comorbidities with a high or prohibitive risk for surgical intervention. Studies with a large study population and long-term outcomes are limited. Furthermore, many transcatheter devices for TMVI are in a preclinical study evolution or in the study design. The recruitment of patients for TMVI plays a crucial role to increase the number of patients who will undergo TMVI in order to derive any safe conclusions about the effectiveness and long-term durability of these devices. On the other hand, the valve-in-valve implantation in the degenerated prosthetic valve or ring annuloplasty was reported in the literature with acceptable short- and mid-term results [9,11,12]. In this review, we present the current studies with reported outcomes after TMVI in the last few years. We present in Table 1 the baseline characteristics, indications and the most common post-procedural complications from these studies, while in Table 2, the outcomes of patients who underwent TMVI are presented.

Table 1. Baseline characteristics of patients, indications for TMVI and the most common post-procedural complications after TVMI. VIV = valve-in-valve; VIR = valve-in-ring; VIM = valve-in-mitral valve calcification; N/A = not applicable; MAC = mitral annular calcification; MR = mitral valve regurgitation; MS = mitral stenosis; MD = mixed disease; NYHA class = New York Heart Association Classification; IQR = interquartile range.

Authors	Device	Study Population, Number of Patients	Age, Years Old	Gender (Female), %	Pre-Procedural NYHA Class III or III-IV, %	Indications	Post-TMVI Cerebrovascular Accident, %	Post-TMVI Permanent Pacemaker Implantation, %	Success Implantation, %
Wild et al. [24]	Tendyne™	108	Mean 75.5 ± 7	43	86	Severe MR	N/A	N/A	96
Gössl et al. [25]	Tendyne™	20	Mean 78 ± 6	55	90	MR in 11 pts MAC in 9 pts	5	N/A	95
Muller et al. [26]	Tendyne™	100	Mean 74.7 ± 8.0	31	66	Sever MR	N/A	N/A	97
Ussia et al. [27]	CardiAQ™	1	72	0	100	Severe MR	0	0	100
Sondergaard et al. [28]	CardiAQ™	3	Mean 82.3	33	100	Severe MR	0	N/A	100
Ludwig et al. [29]	Tendyne™ and Tiara™	7 and 4	Mean 73.4	72.7	100	Severe MR	0	0	100
Bapat et al. [30]	Intrepid™	50	Mean 73 ± 9	42	86	Severe MR	4	0	98
Zahr et al. [31]	Intrepid™	15	Median 80 (IQR:73–84)	13	67	Severe MR	0	0	93.3
Web et al. [32]	Sapien M3	10	Mean 76.1 ± 5.5	50	100	Severe MR	0	0	100
Eleid et al. [33]	Sapien, Sapien XT, Sapien 3 THV	Total = 87 VIV = 60 VIR = 15 VIM = 12	Mean 75 ± 11 72 ± 8 79 ± 9	57 60 42	100	Sever MR and MAC	N/A	N/A	Overall = 90
Guerrero et al. [34]	Sapien, Sapien XT, Sapien3	Total = 903 VIV = 680 VIR = 123 VIM = 100	Median 76 73 77	Overall = 59 59.9 48 69	89	Sever MR and MAC	1.9	1.2	Overall = 78.7
Whisenant et al. [19]	Sapien 3 THV	1529 (VIV)	Mean 73.3 ± 11.8	59.1	86	Prosthetic valve MS, MR, MD	0.7	0	96.8

Table 2. Studies with outcomes during follow-up included in review. VIV = valve-in-valve; VIR = valve-in-ring; VIM = valve-in-mitral valve calcification; N/A = not applicable.

Authors	Device	Study Period, Years	Study Population, Number of Patients	In-Hospital Mortality, %	1-Year Mortality, %	2-Years Mortality, %
Wild et al. [24]	Tendyne™	2020–2021	108	12	N/A	N/A
Gössl et al. [25]	Tendyne™	2018–2019	20	5	40	N/A
Muller et al. [26]	Tendyne™	2014–2017	100	6	26	39
Ussia et al. [27]	CardiAQ™	2016	1	0	N/A	N/A
Sondergaard et al. [28]	CardiAQ™	2015	3	33	N/A	N/A
Ludwig et al. [29]	Tendyne™ and Tiara™	2016–2020	7 and 4	0	33	N/A
Bapat et al. [30]	Intrepid™	2018	50	14	24	N/A
Zahr et al. [31]	Intrepid™	2020–2021	15	0	N/A	N/A
Web et al. [32]	Sapien M3	2017–2018	10	0	N/A	N/A
Eleid et al. [33]	Sapien, Sapien XT, Sapien 3 THV	2014–2017	87 (VIV, VIR, VIM)	6	32 (VIM) 14 (VIV, VIR)	N/A
Guerrero et al. [34]	Sapien, Sapien XT, Sapien3	2013–2017	903 (VIV, VIR, VIM)	18 (VIM) 6.3 (VIV) 9 (VIR)	N/A	N/A
Whisenant et al. [19]	Sapien 3 THV	2015–2019	1529 (VIV)	5.4	16.7	N/A

Recently, the Tendyne Mitral Valve system for TMVI has received a CE mark for the treatment of patients with MV pathologies. Wild et al. reported results from a multicenter study, which included 108 surgical high risk patients with symptomatic MV treated by the Tendyne Mitral Valve system [24]. The majority of patients were readmitted to the hospital due to heart failure and most of them had pre-procedure NYHA class III-IV. The authors reported that the in-hospital mortality was 8%, in-hospital cerebrovascular events were 3%, major bleeding was 11%, valve thrombosis was 1%, permanent pacemaker (PPM) implantation was 2%, sepsis was observed at 10% and acute kidney injury requiring dialysis was 5%. Two patients died peri-procedurally. A total of 64 (66%) patients were discharged at home, with the remaining being transferred to other hospitals or rehabilitation centers [24]; meanwhile, the 30 day mortality was 12%. In addition, the authors reported that during the median follow-up of 50 days, 73% of patients were NYHA functional class I or II ($p < 0.001$), as this compared to pre-TMVI. Gössl et al. published the results after the same mitral valve device implantation in 20 patients [25]. No procedural mortality was reported, while the 30-day mortality and the one-year all-cause mortality was 5% and 40%, respectively. During the one-year follow-up, six patients (31%) were re-admitted for hospitalization due to HF, and the NYHA functional class was upgraded in 11 patients who were alive after one year. Muller at al., in 2021, presents the outcomes after the Tendyne mitral valve implantation at 2 years [26]. This multicenter study included 100 patients with the severe MR of native MV, and the study period was 2014–2017. The study was a clinical trial titled, "Expanded Clinical Study of the Tendyne Mitral Valve System". At the one- and two-year follow-up, the all-cause mortality was 26% and 39%, respectively, while the post-procedural neurological complications, including TIA and stroke, at 1- and 2-year follow-ups, were 6% and 9%, respectively. PPM implantation incidence at the 1- and 2-year follow-up was 7% and 8%, respectively. The thrombosis of the prosthetic valve was observed in 6% of patients during the 2-year follow-up. The most common device related to an adverse event during the 2-year follow-up was the paravalvular leak in 9%.

CardiAQ-Edwards TMVR System was another prosthetic mitral valve, which was used for the treatment of advanced MV pathologies via the transfemoral approach [27]. Ussia et al. presented their results after a first and second-generation CardiAQ mitral valve bioprosthesis implantation in a patient with severe MR. The patient survived 30-days after the implantation at NYHA class I. In 2016, Sondergaard et al. presented their results after CardiAQ implantation in three patients, and one of them died in hospital [28].

The first in-man implantation, the Tiara TMVR system, was described by Cheung et al. in 2014 [35]. Ludwig at al. presented their results after implantation with the following two devices, the Tendyne TMVR system and Tiara™ [29]. In four patients, the Tiara prosthetic valve was implanted and no procedural or in hospital mortality was observed. Stroke, prosthetic valve thrombosis, myocardial infarction or re-intervention was not observed after 30 days. In this report, the authors demonstrated that the mortality rate after 3, 6 and 12 months was 10, 22.2 and 33.3%, respectively, but unfortunately they did not focus on mortality rate with regards to the specific type of mitral valve prosthesis. The clinical trial, the Tiara™ Transcatheter Mitral Valve Replacement Study (TIARA-II), was started in 2017, and the estimated date for completion will be in 2026.

Bapat et al. presented the early experience after the Medtronic Intrepid™ Transcatheter Mitral Valve Replacement System implantation in 50 patients in the context of the Intrepid Global Pilot Study Investigators [30]. Most of the patients had secondary MR (72% of patients). The prosthetic valve was implanted transapically. A successful implantation was achieved in 98% of patients. The median procedure time was 100 min and in 5% of patients an intra-aortic balloon pump was placed. The median follow-up of patients was 173 days, and the 30-day mortality was 14%. The all-cause mortality during follow-up was 9.8%. After procedure (>30 days), the rehospitalization for heart failure was recorded in 19.5% of patients. Reoperation for bleeding immediately after operation was performed in five patients, while postoperative neurological complications after implantation and during follow-up (including stroke) were observed in 6.4% of patients. During the 30-day follow-up, the NYHA class was upgraded for the functional class I and II in 79% of patients. The pulmonary artery systolic pressure was reduced post-procedural ($p < 0.001$). Zahr et al. reported the 30-day outcome of 15 patients, who were treated for moderate to severe or severe MR by the Intrepid™ Transcatheter Mitral Valve Replacement System and transfemoral approach [31]. The study period was from 2020 to 2021 and the 35-F-delivered system was used for the transfemoral valve implantation. The patient clinical status and echocardiography were followed up at 30-days. The median age of the study population was 80 years old, and 53% of the patients have undergone cardiac surgery in the past. The preoperative primary MR was recorded in 67% of patients. No deaths, postoperative neurological complications, re-interventions and PPM implantation was observed at the 30-day post-procedural follow-up period, while major or worse bleeding was recorded in 47% of patients. In 15% of patients, moderate LVOT obstruction was observed.

The first in-human implantation outcomes with the new TMVI devices (Edwards Sapien M3, Edwards Lifesciences, Irvine, CA, USA) presented by Webb et al. [32]. The prosthetic valve was implanted by the transfemoral approach. The study period was from 2017 until 2018 and 10 patients were included. The mean age was 76.1 years old and 50% of the patients were men. Degenerative and secondary MR was observed in 40 and 40% of patients, respectively. The mortality and stroke in the first 30 days after implantation was 0%. LVOT obstruction was not recognized clinically or echocardiogrphically during or after implantation.

The transcatheter mitral valve implantation in patients with the degenerated prosthetic valve and previously failed surgical repair is the most common practice for prosthetic valve implantation by transcatheter methods. In addition, these patients are poor candidates for reoperation due to a high perioperative risk for complication and deaths [19,33,34,36]. Eleid et al. presented a study of the early outcomes (1-year) of a multi-center study of 87 patients who underwent TMVI for failed mitral bioprothesis in 60 patients [valve-in-valve (VIV)], ring annuloplasty [valve-in-ring (VIR)] and severe mitral annular calcification [valve in mitral annular calcification (VMAC)] in 60, 15 and 12 patients, respectively [33]. The study period was 2014–2017 and the balloon-expandable SAPIEN, SAPIEN XT, or SAPIEN 3 THV (Edwards Lifesciences, Irvine, California) were used for TMVI. The mean age of patients was 75 years old, and procedural success was 90%. TMVI was performed by trans-septal/transfemoral and transapical methods in 84 and 3 patients, respectively, while the total peri-procedure mortality was 5%. The LVOT obstruction was observed in 9% of patients and most frequently occurred in the valve-in ring (20%) group. Prosthetic valve thrombosis was diagnosed in two patients. The 30-day mortality overall was 6%. The mean follow-up in the VIV and VIR was 283 and 309 days, respectively. The survival rate at the 1-year follow-up in VIV, VIR and VMAC were 86%, 82% and 57%, respectively. The predictor factor for the LVOT obstruction was a higher LVEF and most of the patients were treated conservatively. Guerrero et al. reported 30-day outcomes of TMVI for patients who underwent VIV, VIR and VMAC [34]. The study period was 2013–2017. It was a retrospective analysis of the national database of USA and included 903 patients from 127 hospitals. Most of these patients underwent VIV = 680 patients, and SAPIEN 3 valve (Edwards Lifesciences, Irvine, CA, USA) was the most common prosthetic valve. The 30-day mortality in the study population was 10.1% and it was higher in the VMAC group (21.8%). The accesses for TMVI were transapical and transseptal methods in 44.8% and 43.1%, respectively. IABP insertion was needed in 3.2% of overall patients, while the PPM insertion was 1.2%. The incidence of postoperative neurological complications at the 30-day follow-up was 1.7% and myocardial infarction was 0.5%. Moreover, knowledge about TMVI in patients with failed mitral bioprothesis was reported by Whisenant et al. [19]. Their research focused on 1-year outcomes of patients who underwent VIV for failed mitral prosthesis. The SAPIEN 3 valve (Edwards Lifesciences, Irvine, CA) was used for TMVI. The study period was from 2015 until 2019 and included patients. The transseptal approach was the most common access for TMVI (86.7%). The patients' age was 73.3 years old and prosthetic mitral valve stenosis was the most common pathology (55.4%). The most commonly implanted SAPIEN 3 size was 29-mm (56%). At 30 days, the all-cause mortality, stroke and PPM implantation were 5.4%, 1.1% and 1.4%, respectively. Meanwhile, during the 1-year follow-up, the all-cause mortality, stroke, PPM implantation, mitral valve re-intervention and device thrombosis were 16.7%, 3.3%, 2.1%, 0.8% and 0.5%, respectively.

4. Conclusions

Surgical mitral valve replacement or repair remain the gold standard technique for patients with primary MR therapy, while the patients with secondary MR, severe MAC, degenerated prosthetic mitral valve and failed MVr (surgically or transcatheter) remain in the gray zone regarding the appropriate choice for invasive or non-invasive therapy. The rising numbers of elderly patients with coexisting complex comorbidities with advanced mitral valve pathologies creates a large population not suitable for surgical operation. Untreated progressive mitral valve diseases negatively affect the quality of life, morbidity and survival rate of these patients. Alternative options for therapy are transcatheter mitral valve therapy, including the edge-to-edge technique, percutaneous mitral ring annuloplasty and TMVI. Meanwhile, in patients with secondary (functional) moderate to severe or severe MR, the MitrClip have promising results; the patients with severe MAC, degenerated mitral bioprothesis and severe primary MR with LV dysfunction consist of practice-inoperable patients, and probably need to be treated conservatively. TMVI can cover the gap for making a decision for an appropriate therapy in these patients. Although the 30-day mortality after TMVI is 0–10%, more studies with larger-studied populations are required in order to derive safe conclusions about the effectiveness of TMVI therapy and the durability of new devices in current clinical practice.

Author Contributions: All authors contributed equally in carrying out the research and writing the manuscript. All authors have read and agreed to the published version of the manuscript.

Funding: This research received no external funding.

Institutional Review Board Statement: Ethical review and approval were waived for this study due to the nature of this study (review).

Informed Consent Statement: Not applicable.

Data Availability Statement: Not applicable.

Conflicts of Interest: The authors declare no conflict of interest.

References

1. Writing Committee Members; Otto, C.M.; Nishimura, R.A.; Bonow, R.O.; Carabello, B.A.; Erwin, J.P., 3rd; Gentile, F.; Jneid, H.; Krieger, E.V.; Mack, M.; et al. 2020 ACC/AHA Guideline for the Management of Patients with Valvular Heart Diseass: A Report of the American College of Cardiology/American Heart Association Joint Committee on Clinical Practice Guidelines. *J. Am. Coll. Cardiol.* **2021**, *77*, e25–e197. [CrossRef] [PubMed]
2. Beyersdorf, F.; Vahanian, A.; Milojevic, M.; Praz, F.; Baldus, S.; Bauersachs, J.; Capodanno, D.; Conradi, L.; De Bonis, M.; De Paulis, R.; et al. 2021 ESC/EACTS Guidelines for the management of valvular heart disease. *Eur. J. Cardio-Thoracic Surg.* **2021**, *60*, 727–800. [CrossRef] [PubMed]
3. Izumi, C.; Eishi, K.; Ashihara, K.; Arita, T.; Otsuji, Y.; Kunihara, T.; Komiya, T.; Shibata, T.; Seo, Y.; Daimon, M.; et al. JCS/JSCS/JATS/JSVS 2020 Guidelines on the Management of Valvular Heart Disease. *Circ. J.* **2020**, *84*, 2037–2119. [CrossRef] [PubMed]
4. Godino, C.; Scotti, A.; Taramasso, M.; Adamo, M.; Russo, M.; Chiarito, M.; Melillo, F.; Beneduce, A.; Pivato, C.A.; Arrigoni, L.; et al. Two-year cardiac mortality after MitraClip treatment of functional mitral regurgitation in ischemic and non-ischemic dilated cardiomyopathy. *Int. J. Cardiol.* **2018**, *269*, 33–39. [CrossRef]
5. Messika-Zeitoun, D.; Nickenig, G.; Latib, A.; Kuck, K.-H.; Baldus, S.; Schueler, R.; La Canna, G.; Agricola, E.; Kreidel, F.; Huntgeburth, M.; et al. Transcatheter mitral valve repair for functional mitral regurgitation using the Cardioband system: 1 year outcomes. *Eur. Heart J.* **2018**, *40*, 466–472. [CrossRef] [PubMed]
6. Guadagnoli, A.F.; De Carlo, C.; Maisano, F.; Ho, E.; Saccocci, M.; Cuevas, O.; Luciani, M.; Kuwata, S.; Nietlispach, F.; Taramasso, M. Cardioband system as a treatment for functional mitral regurgitation. *Expert Rev. Med. Devices* **2018**, *15*, 415–421. [CrossRef]
7. Dahle, G. Current Devices in TMVI and Their Limitations: Focus on Tendyne. *Front. Cardiovasc. Med.* **2020**, *7*, 592909. [CrossRef]

8. Werner, N.; Kilkowski, C.; Sutor, D.; Weisse, U.; Schneider, S.; Zahn, R. Transcatheter Mitral Valve Implantation (TMVI) Using Edwards SAPIEN 3 Prostheses in Patients at Very High or Prohibitive Surgical Risk: A Single-Center Experience. *J. Interv. Cardiol.* **2020**, *2020*, 9485247. [CrossRef]
9. Khan, M.Z.; Zahid, S.; Kichloo, A.; Jamal, S.; Minhas, A.M.K.; Ullah, W.; Sattar, Y.; Balla, S. Redo Surgical Mitral Valve Replacement Versus Transcatheter Mitral Valve in Valve from the National Inpatient Sample. *J. Am. Heart Assoc.* **2021**, *10*, e020948. [CrossRef]
10. Lima, F.V.; Kolte, D.; Rofeberg, V.; Molino, J.; Zhang, Z.; Elmariah, S.; Aronow, H.D.; Abbott, J.D.; Ben Assa, E.; Khera, S.; et al. Thirty-day readmissions after transcatheter versus surgical mitral valve repair in high-risk patients with mitral regurgitation: Analysis of the 2014–2015 Nationwide readmissions databases. *Catheter. Cardiovasc. Interv.* **2019**, *96*, 664–674. [CrossRef]
11. Simard, T.; Lloyd, J.; Crestanello, J.; Thaden, J.J.; Alkhouli, M.; Guerrero, M.; Rihal, C.S.; Eleid, M.F. Five-year outcomes of transcatheter mitral valve implantation and redo surgery for mitral prosthesis degeneration. *Catheter. Cardiovasc. Interv.* **2022**, *99*, 1659–1665. [CrossRef] [PubMed]
12. Martinez-Gomez, E.; McInerney, A.; Tirado-Conte, G.; Agustin, J.A.; Jimenez-Quevedo, P.; Escudero, A.; Osinalde, E.P.; Viana-Tejedor, A.; Goirigolzarri, J.; Marroquin, L.; et al. Percutaneous mitral valve repair with MitraClip device in hemodynamically unstable patients: A systematic review. *Catheter. Cardiovasc. Interv.* **2021**, *98*, E617–E625. [CrossRef]
13. Søndergaard, L.; De Backer, O.; Franzen, O.W.; Holme, S.J.; Ihlemann, N.; Vejlstrup, N.G.; Hansen, P.B.; Quadri, A. First-in-Human Case of Transfemoral CardiAQ Mitral Valve Implantation. *Circ. Cardiovasc. Interv.* **2015**, *8*, e002135. [CrossRef] [PubMed]
14. Al-Hijji, M.A.; ElHajj, S.; El Sabbagh, A.; Alkhouli, M.A.; Crestanello, J.; Eleid, M.F.; Rihal, C.; Guerrero, M. Temporal outcomes of transcatheter mitral valve replacement in native mitral valve disease with annular calcification. *Catheter. Cardiovasc. Interv.* **2021**, *98*, E602–E609. [CrossRef] [PubMed]
15. Enta, Y.; Nakamura, M. Transcatheter mitral valve replacement. *J. Cardiol.* **2020**, *77*, 555–564. [CrossRef]
16. Obadia, J.-F.; Messika-Zeitoun, D.; Leurent, G.; Iung, B.; Bonnet, G.; Piriou, N.; Lefèvre, T.; Piot, C.; Rouleau, F.; Carrié, D.; et al. Percutaneous Repair or Medical Treatment for Secondary Mitral Regurgitation. *N. Engl. J. Med.* **2018**, *379*, 2297–2306. [CrossRef]
17. Iung, B.; Armoiry, X.; Vahanian, A.; Boutitie, F.; Mewton, N.; Trochu, J.; Lefèvre, T.; Messika-Zeitoun, D.; Guerin, P.; Cormier, B.; et al. Percutaneous repair or medical treatment for secondary mitral regurgitation: Outcomes at 2 years. *Eur. J. Heart Fail.* **2019**, *21*, 1619–1627. [CrossRef]
18. Stone, G.W.; Lindenfeld, J.; Abraham, W.T.; Kar, S.; Lim, D.S.; Mishell, J.M.; Whisenant, B.; Grayburn, P.A.; Rinaldi, M.; Kapadia, S.R.; et al. Transcatheter Mitral-Valve Repair in Patients with Heart Failure. *N. Engl. J. Med.* **2018**, *379*, 2307–2318. [CrossRef]
19. Whisenant, B.; Kapadia, S.R.; Eleid, M.F.; Kodali, S.K.; McCabe, J.M.; Krishnaswamy, A.; Morse, M.; Smalling, R.W.; Reisman, M.; Mack, M.; et al. One-Year Outcomes of Mitral Valve-in-Valve Using the SAPIEN 3 Transcatheter Heart Valve. *JAMA Cardiol.* **2020**, *5*, 1245–1252. [CrossRef]
20. Zhang, B.; Li, M.; Kang, Y.; Xing, L.; Zhang, Y. Comparison of different transcatheter interventions for treatment of mitral regurgitation: A protocol for a network meta-analysis. *Medicine* **2020**, *99*, e23623. [CrossRef]
21. Sorajja, P.; Moat, N.; Badhwar, V.; Walters, D.; Paone, G.; Bethea, B.; Bae, R.; Dahle, G.; Mumtaz, M.; Grayburn, P.; et al. Initial Feasibility Study of a New Transcatheter Mitral Prosthesis: The First 100 Patients. *J. Am. Coll. Cardiol.* **2019**, *73*, 1250–1260. [CrossRef] [PubMed]
22. Perez-Camargo, D.; Chen, M.; Taramasso, M. Devices for transcatheter mitral valve repair: Current technology and a glimpse into the future. *Expert Rev. Med. Devices* **2021**, *18*, 609–628. [CrossRef] [PubMed]
23. Goode, D.; Dhaliwal, R.; Mohammadi, H. Transcatheter Mitral Valve Replacement: State of the Art. *Cardiovasc. Eng. Technol.* **2020**, *11*, 229–253. [CrossRef] [PubMed]
24. Wild, M.G.; Kreidel, F.; Hell, M.M.; Praz, F.; Mach, M.; Adam, M.; Reineke, D.; Ruge, H.; Ludwig, S.; Conradi, L.; et al. Transapical mitral valve implantation for treatment of symptomatic mitral valve disease: A real-world multicentre experience. *Eur. J. Heart Fail.* **2022**, *24*, 899–907. [CrossRef] [PubMed]
25. Gössl, M.; Thourani, V.; Babaliaros, V.; Conradi, L.; Chehab, B.; Dumonteil, N.; Badhwar, V.; Rizik, D.; Sun, B.; Bae, R.; et al. Early outcomes of transcatheter mitral valve replacement with the Tendyne system in severe mitral annular calcification. *EuroIntervention* **2022**, *17*, 1523–1531. [CrossRef]
26. Muller, D.W.; Sorajja, P.; Duncan, A.; Bethea, B.; Dahle, G.; Grayburn, P.; Babaliaros, V.; Guerrero, M.; Thourani, V.H.; Bedogni, F.; et al. 2-Year Outcomes of Transcatheter Mitral Valve Replacement in Patients with Severe Symptomatic Mitral Regurgitation. *J. Am. Coll. Cardiol.* **2021**, *78*, 1847–1859. [CrossRef]
27. Ussia, G.P.; Quadri, A.; Cammalleri, V.; De Vico, P.; Muscoli, S.; Marchei, M.; Ruvolo, G.; Sondergaard, L.; Romeo, F. Percutaneous transfemoral-transseptal implantation of a second-generation CardiAQ™ mitral valve bioprosthesis: First procedure description and 30-day follow-up. *EuroIntervention* **2016**, *11*, 1126–1151. [CrossRef]
28. Sondergaard, L.; Brooks, M.; Ihlemann, N.; Jonsson, A.; Holme, S.; Tang, M.; Terp, K.; Quadri, A. Transcatheter mitral valve implantation via transapical approach: An early experience. *Eur. J. Cardio-Thoracic Surg.* **2015**, *48*, 873–878, discussion 877–878. [CrossRef]
29. Ludwig, S.; Kalbacher, D.; Schofer, N.; Schäfer, A.; Koell, B.; Seiffert, M.; Schirmer, J.; Westermann, D.; Reichenspurner, H.; Blankenberg, S.; et al. Early results of a real-world series with two transapical transcatheter mitral valve replacement devices. *Clin. Res. Cardiol.* **2020**, *110*, 411–420. [CrossRef]
30. Bapat, V.; Rajagopal, V.; Meduri, C.; Farivar, R.S.; Walton, A.; Duffy, S.J.; Gooley, R.; Almeida, A.; Reardon, M.J.; Kleiman, N.S.; et al. Early Experience with New Transcatheter Mitral Valve Replacement. *J. Am. Coll. Cardiol.* **2017**, *71*, 12–21. [CrossRef]

31. Zahr, F.; Song, H.K.; Chadderdon, S.M.; Gada, H.; Mumtaz, M.; Byrne, T.; Kirshner, M.; Bajwa, T.; Weiss, E.; Kodali, S.; et al. 30-Day Outcomes Following Transfemoral Transseptal Transcatheter Mitral Valve Replacement. *JACC Cardiovasc. Interv.* **2021**, *15*, 80–89. [CrossRef] [PubMed]
32. Webb, J.G.; Murdoch, D.J.; Boone, R.H.; Moss, R.; Attinger-Toller, A.; Blanke, P.; Cheung, A.; Hensey, M.; Leipsic, J.; Ong, K.; et al. Percutaneous Transcatheter Mitral Valve Replacement: First-in-Human Experience Tableith a New Transseptal System. *J. Am. Coll. Cardiol.* **2019**, *73*, 1239–1246. [CrossRef] [PubMed]
33. Eleid, M.F.; Whisenant, B.K.; Cabalka, A.K.; Williams, M.R.; Nejjari, M.; Attias, D.; Fam, N.; Amoroso, N.; Foley, T.A.; Pollak, P.M.; et al. Early Outcomes of Percutaneous Transvenous Transseptal Transcatheter Valve Implantation in Failed Bioprosthetic Mitral Valves, Ring Annuloplasty, and Severe Mitral Annular Calcification. *JACC Cardiovasc. Interv.* **2017**, *10*, 1932–1942. [CrossRef]
34. Guerrero, M.; Vemulapalli, S.; Xiang, Q.; Wang, D.D.; Eleid, M.; Cabalka, A.K.; Sandhu, G.; Salinger, M.; Russell, H.; Greenbaum, A.; et al. Thirty-Day Outcomes of Transcatheter Mitral Valve Replacement for Degenerated Mitral Bioprostheses (Valve-in-Valve), Failed Surgical Rings (Valve-in-Ring), and Native Valve with Severe Mitral Annular Calcification (Valve-in-Mitral Annular Calcification) in the United States: Data From the Society of Thoracic Surgeons/American College of Cardiology/Transcatheter Valve Therapy Registry. *Circ. Cardiovasc. Interv.* **2020**, *13*, e008425. [CrossRef] [PubMed]
35. Cheung, A.; Webb, J.; Verheye, S.; Moss, R.; Boone, R.; Leipsic, J.; Ree, R.; Banai, S. Short-Term Results of Transapical Transcatheter Mitral Valve Implantation for Mitral Regurgitation. *J. Am. Coll. Cardiol.* **2014**, *64*, 1814–1819. [CrossRef] [PubMed]
36. Cheung, A.; Webb, J.G.; Barbanti, M.; Freeman, M.; Binder, R.K.; Thompson, C.; Wood, D.A.; Ye, J. 5-Year experience with transcatheter transapical mitral valve-in-valve implantation for bioprosthetic valve dysfunction. *J. Am. Coll. Cardiol.* **2013**, *61*, 1759–1766. [CrossRef] [PubMed]

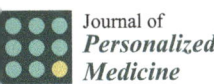

Systematic Review

Cerebral Aneurysms Caused by Atrial Myxoma—A Systematic Review of the Literature

Justyna Chojdak-Łukasiewicz, Sławomir Budrewicz and Marta Waliszewska-Prosół *

Department of Neurology, Wroclaw Medical University, 50-556 Wroclaw, Poland
* Correspondence: marta.waliszewska-prosol@umw.edu.pl; Tel.: +48-71-734-3100; Fax: +48-71-734-3109

Abstract: Background: The association between cerebral aneurysms and left atrial myxoma is known but rare. We described its pathogenesis, clinical presentation, diagnostic findings and treatment using a systemic review of the literature. **Methods**: MEDLINE via PubMed was searched for articles published until August 2022 using the keywords "atrial myxoma", "cardiac myxoma" and "cerebral aneurysm". **Results**: In this review, 55 patients with multiple myxomas aneurysms were analyzed, and 65% were women. The average age when aneurysms were diagnosed was 42.5 ± 15.81; most patients were less than 60 years old (86%). Aneurysms could be found before the diagnosis, at the same time as cardiac myxoma, or even 25 years after resection of the atrial mass. In our review, the mean time to diagnoses was 4.5 years. Our review estimates that the most common symptoms were vascular incidents (25%) and seizures (14.3%). In 15 cases, variable headaches were reported. Regarding management strategies, 57% cases were managed conservatively as the primary choice. **Conclusions**: Although cerebral aneurysms caused by atrial myxoma are rare, the long-term consequences can be serious and patients should be monitored.

Keywords: atrial myxoma; cerebral aneurysm; metastatic aneurysm; headache; cardiac tumors

1. Introduction

Cardiac myxomas (CM) are the most common benign "cardiac" tumors, accounting for up to 30–50% of all primary heart tumors [1]. The incidence is approximately 0.5–1 cases per 1,000,000 population per year [2]. About 75% concern the left atrium of the heart [3], and 18% originate in the right atrium; biatrial myxomas are rare and account for less than 2.5% of all cardiac myxomas. Myxomas are particularly frequent from the third to the sixth decades of life; the ratio women: men varies from 2:1 to 3:1. CM are diagnosed based on clinical examination and tests such as electrocardiography (ECG), transthoracic echocardiogram (TTE), transesophageal echocardiogram (TEE), chest computed tomography (CT) or magnetic resonance imaging (MRI) and cardiac MRI [4].

Most cardiac myxomas present with constitutional, embolic and obstructive manifestations. Younger and male patients have more neurologic symptoms, and female patients have more systemic symptoms. These can cause many neurological complications, including systemic embolism, cerebral infarction, cerebral cavernous malformations and intracranial aneurysms [5]. Myxoma-related aneurysms are always multiple and in most cases have a fusiform-shape.

Left atrial myxomas are considered curable by complete resection and give excellent results in long-term follow-up. Surgical excision remains the treatment of choice for cardiac myxoma. Early diagnosis and intervention is desirable because of the persistent risk of brain metastases and aneurysms. However, incomplete resection, multifocal tumors and embolism caused by tumors are important factors in its recurrence and complications [3,6]. Currently, our understanding of cerebral aneurysms caused by atrial myxoma is based mainly on case reports.

Citation: Chojdak-Łukasiewicz, J.; Budrewicz, S.; Waliszewska-Prosół, M. Cerebral Aneurysms Caused by Atrial Myxoma—A Systematic Review of the Literature. *J. Pers. Med.* **2023**, *13*, 8. https://doi.org/10.3390/jpm13010008

Academic Editor: Georgios Samanidis

Received: 11 November 2022
Revised: 11 December 2022
Accepted: 19 December 2022
Published: 21 December 2022

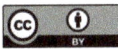

Copyright: © 2022 by the authors. Licensee MDPI, Basel, Switzerland. This article is an open access article distributed under the terms and conditions of the Creative Commons Attribution (CC BY) license (https://creativecommons.org/licenses/by/4.0/).

This systemic review of the literature aimed to provide an exhaustive summary of available case reports evaluating medical history, clinical, diagnostic and therapeutic methods in patients with cerebral aneurysms caused by atrial myxoma.

2. Methods

JCŁ and MWP performed an independent online search in accordance with PRISMA guidelines [7] using the following combination of keywords: "atrial" and "cardiac" and "myxoma" and "cerebral" and "aneurysm" or "myxomatosus" and "cerebral" and "aneurysm".

We considered publication records from MEDLINE and ERIC databases until August 2022. In addition, the reference lists from eligible publications were searched. All discrepancies were resolved by discussing the results of the preliminary search with a third reviewer (SB) (Figure 1).

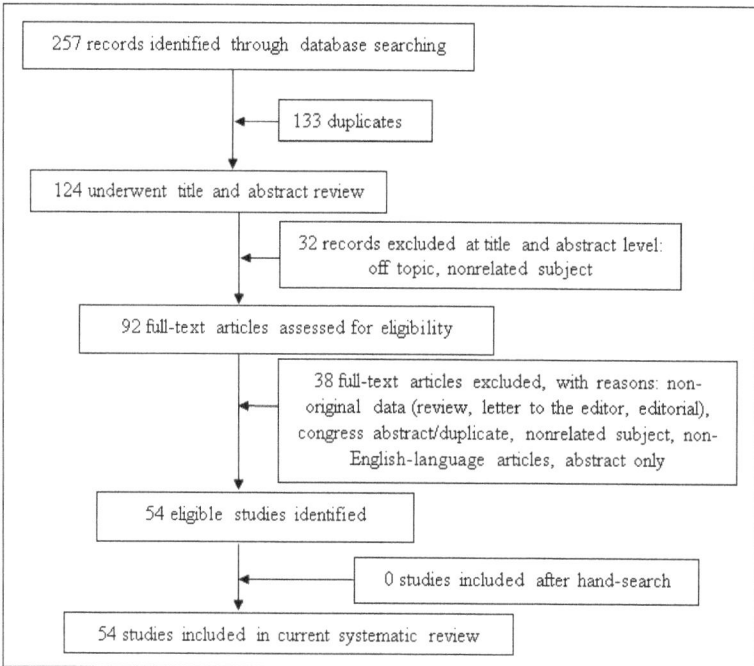

Figure 1. Flow chart of study selection.

A total of 257 records were identified and screened separately by the authors. Then, these record lists were double read by both analysts and 92 abstracts were found to be relevant to the subject. Each researcher worked independently and prepared their own list of relevant full-text manuscripts. Both lists were compared and 54 publications were found to be the most relevant to the study and included in this review. The exclusion criteria were non-English-language articles, conference papers and abstract only.

3. Results

We found 54 case report articles describing 55 patients. All cases are illustrated in Table 1. We did not find any article about type case series or an original work on a larger group of patients. The group consisted of 35 women (64%) and 20 men (36%). The average age when aneurysms were diagnosed was 42.5 ± 15.81 years (the age varied from 11 to 69 years) and 46 of the patients were less than 60 years old (84%).

Table 1. Overview of cases of cerebral aneurysms in atrial myxoma from the literature.

	Author	Case	Clinical Presentation	Atrial Myxoma History	Radiological Findings	Cardiological Treatment	Aneurysm Procedure
1.	Airohimi et al. [8]	37-year-old woman	thunderclap headache with right-sided ptosis	left atrial myxoma diagnosed at the same time	CTA—right posterior communicating artery aneurysm	open heart surgery	right posterior communicating aneurysm clipping
2.	Asranna et al. [9]	57-year-old woman	secondary generalized seizures	left atrial myxoma resection 1 year earlier	DSA—multiple fusiform aneurysms involving the left middle cerebral artery (MCA) M3 segment and angular branch	open heart surgery	conservative
3.	Ashalatha et al. [10]	54-year-old man	left focal motor seizures with secondary generalization	left atrial myxoma 6 months earlier	DSA—multiple, small, distal, fusiform aneurysms along both middle and anterior cerebral arteries	open heart surgery	conservative
4.	Baikoussis et al. [11]	72-year-old woman	vertigo and collapse with loss of consciousness	left atrial myxoma diagnosed at the same time	MR—multiple cerebral mycotic aneurysms of various dimensions and a large cyst, as a result of a previous hemorrhage	open heart surgery	embolization of the large central aneurysms
5.	Bernet et al. [12]	31-year-old woman	general clonic-tonic seizure	left atrial myxoma resection 2 months earlier	CT—multiple frontal and occipital bilateral cerebral aneurysm	open heart surgery	radiation plus chemotherapy
6.	Branscheidt et al. [13]	41-year-old woman	"burning" headaches and increasing fatigue	left atrial myxoma diagnosed at the same time	DSA—multiple fusiform aneurysms	open heart surgery	chemotherapy
7.	Chen et al. [14]	19-year-old woman	seizures without loss of consciousness	left atrial myxoma resection 2 years earlier	DSA—many saccular dilatations on the distal end of the MCA and PCA of both sides	open heart surgery	conservative
8.	Chow et al. [15]	58-year-old woman	loss of consciousness 2 years earlier SAH (external ventricular drainage was executed)	left atrial myxoma without resection	DSA—lobulated aneurysm at the middle cerebral arterial with clipping executed.	open heart surgery	conservative
9.	Desousa et al. [16]	44-year-old woman	left-sided headache, vomiting	left atrial myxoma resection 8 years earlier	carotid angiogram demonstrated progressive narrowing of the left internal carotid artery	open heart surgery	conservative
10.	Eddleman et al. [17]	18-year-old man	episode of scintillations in the right visual field lasting 2 h associated with a headache	left atrial myxoma resection 4 months earlier	DSA—multiple fusiform aneurysms the distal anterior, middle, and posterior circulations	open heart surgery	resection some aneurysm
11.	Ezerioha et al. [18]	73-year-old woman	SAH	left atrial myxoma recognized at the same time	CTA 9-mm lobulated aneurysm at the right middle cerebral artery (MCA) trifurcation and a small 3-mm aneurysm at the left MCA bifurcation	open heart surgery	right frontal pterional craniotomy, evaluation of intracerebral hematoma and clipping of the right MCA aneurysm
12.	Flores et al. [19]	19-year-old woman	right-sided hemiparesis lasting for one hour	left atrial myxoma recognized at the same time	DSA—multiple fusiform cerebral aneurysms affecting several distal branches of both middle cerebral arteries	open heart surgery	conservative
13.	Flores et al. [19]	61-year-old man	acute onset of rotational vertigo and left visual field deficit, stroke 20 years ago	left atrial myxoma recognized at the same time	DSA—multiple fusiform cerebral aneurysms in the left posteroinferior cerebellar artery, two aneurysms in the M2 segment of the right middle cerebral artery	open heart surgery	conservative
14.	Furuya et al. [20]	36-year-old man	sudden attack of generalized convulsive seizures	left atrial myxoma resection 1 year earlier	DSA—multiple fusiform aneurysms at right operculofrontal, central, and angular arteries	open heart surgery	resection aneurysms of the angular artery

Table 1. *Cont.*

	Author	Case	Clinical Presentation	Atrial Myxoma History	Radiological Findings	Cardiological Treatment	Aneurysm Procedure
15.	George et al. [21]	45-year-old woman	transient ischemic attack	left atrial myxoma recognized at the same time	DSA—multiple fusiform aneurysm at the right middle cerebral artery aneurysm	open heart surgery	conservative
16.	Gupta et al. [22]	11-year-old boy	syncope	left atrial myxoma resection 1 year earlier	CT angiography tortuous, dilated and fusiform left MCA and multiple aneurysms in bilateral MCA and both vertebral arteries	open heart surgery	conservative
17.	Herbst et al. [23]	31-year-old man	dizziness, nausea, blurred vision of his left eye, and gait disturbance	left atrial myxoma was discovered at the same moment	DSA—multiple intracranial microaneurysms in peripheral branches of middle, anterior, and posterior cerebral arteries; a few aneurysms were seen in branches of the vertebrobasilar arteries	open heart surgery	conservative
18.	Hau et al. [5]	57-year-old man	confusion and memory loss	left atrial myxoma resection 2 years earlier	CTA—multiple fusiform intracranial aneurysms at left anterior cerebral artery (ACA) A2 segment bifurcation, right middle cerebral artery (MCA) distal M2 segment, cortical branches at frontal and para-central regions, left posterior cerebral artery (PCA) P3 segment, and right occipital cortical branches, with progressive enlargement half-yearly	open heart surgery	stereotactic radiosurgery
19.	Iskandar et al. [24]	69-year-old woman	left arm numbness, weakness, and dysarthria	left atrial recurrent myxoma resection 20 and 15 years earlier	CTA—myxomatous fusiform aneurysms in the right middle cerebral arteries	open heart surgery	conservative
20.	Ivanovic et al. [25]	44-year-old woman	ten months earlier SAH with operation of left PICA aneurysm	left atrial myxoma ten months earlier	DSA—saccular aneurysm arising from the origin of left posterior inferior cerebelli artery	open heart surgery	conservative
21.	Jean et al. [26]	32-year-old woman	transient ischemic attack	left atrial myxoma resection 5 years earlier	DSA—multiple peripheral, fusiform, intracranial aneurysms	open heart surgery	left frontal craniotomy for resection of one of the aneurysms located at the frontal pole
22.	Josephson et al. [27]	33-year-old woman	8 years earlier multiple embolic strokes	left atrial myxoma resection 8 years earlier	MRA—multiple fusiform aneurysms	open heart surgery	conservative
23.	Kim et al. [28]	58-year-old woman	right flank pain for several days 20 years earlier three episodes of stroke with dysarthria and right-sides hemiplegia	left atrial myxoma discovered at the same moment	MRA—multiple fusiform aneurysms of the left distal internal carotid artery, peripheral branch of the right middle cerebral artery, left posterior cerebral artery, and the distal basilar artery	open heart surgery	conservative
24.	Koo et al. [29]	64-year-old woman	dysarthria, generalized weakness, and gait disturbance	left atrial myxoma discovered at the same moment	DSA—multiple fusiform-cerebral aneurysms at distal branches of anterior cerebral arteries (ACA) and middle cerebral arteries (MCA)	open heart surgery	conservative
25.	Krishnan et al. [30]	31-old-year man	two episodes of generalized tonic clonic seizures	left atrial myxoma resection 12 years earlier	CTA—fusiform dilation of bilateral distal anterior cerebral arteries, multiple dilations of distal middle cerebral artery branches on both sides and also aneurysmal dilatation of the distal right posterior cerebral artery	open heart surgery	conservative
26.	Lazarow et al. [31]	52-year-old man	acute right lower extremity weakness and seizures	left atrial myxoma resection 3 years earlier	DSA—diffuse cerebral arterial aneurysms	open heart surgery	left MCA branch was embolized with aneurysm coils

Table 1. *Cont.*

	Author	Case	Clinical Presentation	Atrial Myxoma History	Radiological Findings	Cardiological Treatment	Aneurysm Procedure
27.	Li et al. [32]	27-year-old woman	sudden onset of vertigo, dysarthria and right-sided weakness	left atrial myxoma recognized at the same time	DSA—multiple typical distal fusiform and saccular aneurysms or aneurysmal dilatations in the bilateral internal carotid artery territories	open heart surgery	conservative
28.	Namura et al. [33]	45-year-old man	right hemiparesis 10 years earlier	left atrial myxoma resection after 10 years	DSA—multiple cerebral aneurysms	open heart surgery	conservative
29.	Oguz et al. [34]	40-year-old man	numbness in right arm and blurred vision	left atrial myxoma resection 5 years earlier	DSA—fusiform dilatations in the prefrontal branch of the right MCA, the angular and frontal branches of the left MCA, and the calcarine branch of the left vertebral artery	open heart surgery	conservative
30.	Oomen et al. [35]	40-year-old woman	sensory loss in tongue and face, and word finding difficulty	left atrial myxoma resection 1 year earlier	DSA—micro-aneurysms in the right middle cerebral artery	open heart surgery	conservative
31.	Quan et al. [36]	49-year-old man	acute headache and dizziness	left atrial myxoma recognized at the same time	MRA—multiple small aneurysms	open heart surgery	conservative
32.	Penn et al. [37]	12-year-old boy	a sudden headache, diplopia, gait instability, and speech difficulty	left atrial myxoma recognized at the same time	DSA—numerous a flame-shaped or fusiform dilation on the right internal carotid artery (ICA), a sausage-like fusiform dilation of the right posterior cerebral artery (PCA)	open heart surgery	endovascular treatment
33.	Radoi et al. [38]	45-year-old man	headache, nausea, gait disturbances and weakness of the left extremities	left atrial myxoma resection 16 months earlier	DSA—multiple unruptured intracranial microaneurysms, which were mainly located in the peripheral branches of the left anterior and middle cerebral arteries	open heart surgery	resection the right parietal lesion
34.	Ryou et al. [39]	27-year-old woman	sudden onset dizziness, headache, blurred vision, and tingling sensations in tongue, arm, and the left side of her face	atrial myxoma on both sides, resection 10 years earlier	DSA—revealed multiple fusiform aneurysms in the basilar artery, proximal PICA, left P2 and right P4 segments, temporal branch of the left MCA, and distal branches of the right MCA and ACA	open heart surgery	conservative
35.	Sabolek et al. [40]	43-year-old woman	sudden severe headache, nausea, consciousness disturbances	left atrial myxoma resection 12 years earlier	DSA—fusiform aneurysms of the left anterior cerebral artery, the peripheral branches of the right middle cerebral artery and a giant aneurysm of the basilar artery	open heart surgery	conservative
36.	Saffie et al. [41]	37-year-old man	photopia and headache	left atrial myxoma resection 20 months earlier	DSA—left and right PCA aneurysm	open heart surgery	resection/bypass and clipping
37.	Santillan et al. [42]	68-year-old man	transient ischemic attack	left atrial myxoma resection 14 years earlier	DSA—multiple, fusiform intracranial aneurysms in the anterior and posterior circulation	open heart surgery	conservative
38.	Sato et al. [43]	64-year-old man	right arm weakness and dysarthria	left atrial myxoma recognized at the same time	DSA- multiple, intracranial aneurysms in the anterior and posterior circulation	open heart surgery	conservative
39.	Sedat et al. [44]	50-year-old woman	left hemiplegia	left atrial myxoma resection 5 years earlier	DSA—multiple fusiform aneurysms on the middle, anterior, and posterior cerebral arteries	open heart surgery	radiation

Table 1. Cont.

	Author	Case	Clinical Presentation	Atrial Myxoma History	Radiological Findings	Cardiological Treatment	Aneurysm Procedure
40.	Sørenson et al. [45]	53-year-old man	subacute aphasia and hemiparesis	left atrial myxoma resection 5 years earlier	DSA—multiple intracranial aneurysms, giant fusiform aneurysm of the left middle cerebral artery	open heart surgery	coil embolization
41.	Sriwastara et al. [46]	30-year-old woman	severe right sided headache, weakness of left upper and lower limbs and deviation of angle of mouth to right side with slurring of speech	left atrial myxoma recognized at the same time	CTA saccular aneurysm arising from M2 segment of right MCA	open heart surgery	cerebral aneurysm clipping
42.	Stock et al. [47]	22-year-old woman	none	left atrial myxoma resection 11 years earlier	DSA—aneurysms in both middle cerebral arteries (MCA) and right anterior cerebral artery (ACA)	open heart surgery	conservative
43.	Sveinsson et al. [48]	19-year-old woman	episodic loss of consciousness and right-sided weakness	left atrial myxoma recognized at the same time	DSA—large number of distal well-demarcated fusiform aneurysms	open heart surgery	conservative
44.	Tamuleviciute et al. [49]	29-year-old woman	TIA-like symptoms	left atrial myxoma resection 12 years earlier	DSA—multiple small and fusiform distal aneurysms	open heart surgery	conservative
45.	Vontobel et al. [50]	41-year-old woman	dizziness	left atrial myxoma recognized at the same time	MRA—multiple fusiform aneurysms	open heart surgery	chemotherapy
46.	Waliszewska-Prosół et al. [51]	62-year-old woman	vertigo, tinnitus, headache	left atrial myxoma resection 12 years earlier	DSA—multiple fusiform aneurysms located on peripheral branches of middle (MCA), anterior (ACA), and posterior (PCA) cerebral arteries	open heart surgery	conservative
47.	Waliszewska-Prosół et al. [51]	48-year-old man	a first generalized seizure due to intracranial parenchymal bleeding	left atrial myxoma resection 6 years earlier	SWI—area of intracranial bleeding in the left parietal lobe from a ruptured aneurysm; DSA—multiple fusiform aneurysms located on peripheral branches of the middle, anterior, and posterior cerebral arteries	open heart surgery	conservative
48.	Walker et al. [52]	60-year-old woman	two week history of progressive occipital headache, intermittent visual changes, right facial pain, and imbalance	left atrial myxoma resection 6 years earlier	DSA—large irregular fusiform aneurysms of the proximal SCA bilaterally and a peripheral fusiform aneurysm of a distal posterior right middle cerebral artery branch	open heart surgery	a right pterional craniotomy was undertaken but any component of the aneurysm was suitable for clipping
49.	Wan et al. [3]	39-year-old woman	headache associated with blurred vision	left atrial myxoma resection 1 years earlier	MRA—multiple aneurysms on the bilateral anterior cerebral artery, middle cerebral artery, right posterior cerebral artery and superior cerebellar artery	open heart surgery	clipping of the left ACA arterial aneurysm
50.	Xie et al. [6]	41-year-old man	abnormal behavior and logorrhea	left atrial myxoma recognized at the same time	CTA—large number of cerebral aneurysms mostly on the distal branches of both sides of middle and anterior cerebral artery	open heart surgery	conservative
51.	Xu et al. [53]	46-year-old woman	sudden anesthesia of right upper limb, paroxysmal headache for three months	left atrial myxoma resection 3 years earlier	DSA—multiple fusiform cerebral aneurysms mostly on the middle and some on anterior artery	open heart surgery	conservative
52.	Yilmaz et al. [54]	38-year-old woman	headache, episodes of right sided weakness	left atrial myxoma resection 25 years earlier	DSA—multiple fusiform aneurysms on both carotid artery territories, one of which was a giant aneurysm on the left MCA	open heart surgery	coil embolization of the giant aneurysm

Table 1. Cont.

	Author	Case	Clinical Presentation	Atrial Myxoma History	Radiological Findings	Cardiological Treatment	Aneurysm Procedure
53.	Yoo et al. [55]	20-year-old woman	without symptoms,4 years earlier transient left side motor weakness	left atrial myxoma recognized at the same time	DSA—multiple fusiform cerebral aneurysms, a right MCA fusiform aneurysm was the largest	open heart surgery	M2-M2 bypass surgery
54.	Zeng et al. [56]	60-year-old woman	blunt headache since 2 days	left atrial myxoma resection 2 years earlier	CTA—multiple fusiform aneurysm	open heart surgery	aneurysm was clipped after thrombus dislodgement and angioplasty
55.	Zhang et al. [57]	38-year-old woman	10 days history dizziness and headache	left atrial myxoma and aneurysm recognized at the same time	CTA—two fusiform aneurysms on the left anterior cerebral artery and left posterior cerebral artery	open heart surgery	conservative

CTA—computed tomography angiography; DSA—digital subtraction angiography; CT—computed tomography; MRI—magnetic resonance imaging; MRA—magnetic resonance angiography; SWI—susceptibility weighted imaging; MCA—middle cerebral artery; PICA—posterior inferior cerebellar artery; ICA—internal carotid artery; PCA—posterior cerebral artery; ACA—anterior cerebral artery.

Aneurysms could be found before the diagnosis, at the same time as cardiac myxoma, or even 25 years after resection of atrial mass. In our review, the mean time to diagnoses was 4.5 years. In 1 patient, the myxoma was localized in both atrial, while in the remaining 54 patients—left atrium.

Our review estimates that the most common symptoms were vascular incidents (TIA, stroke), seizures, vertigo or dizziness and loss of consciousness. In 15 cases, variable headaches were reported—most often they had the migraine phenotype with visual disturbances. Three patient presented clinical symptoms typical of subarachnoid hemorrhage and two had no symptoms (Table 2).

Table 2. The most common clinical symptoms.

Clinical Presentation	n (%)	Women:Men	Mean Age
vascular incidents	20 (36.3)	12:8	44.5
headache	15 (27.3)	11:4	40.2
seizures	9 (16.4)	3:6	37.6
vertigo/dizziness	8 (14.5)	6:2	40.1
loss of consciousness	4 (7.3)	4:0	48
subarachnoid hemorrhage	3 (5.5)	3:0	58.3
no symptoms	2 (3.6)	-	-

Based on our analyses, trial myxoma-associated aneurysms are most often localized to the entire area of vascularization, followed by middle cerebral arteries, posterior cerebral arteries, anterior cerebral arteries and finally the basilar artery (Table 3).

Table 3. Location of brain aneurysm.

Location	n	%
multiple—the entire area of vascularization	17	31.1
MCA	16	29.1
MCA + ACA	7	12.7
MCA + PCA	5	9.1
PCA	5	9.1
ACA + PCA	3	5.5
BA	2	3.6

MCA—middle cerebral artery; PCA—posterior cerebral artery; ACA—anterior cerebral artery; BA—basilar artery.

All patients underwent successful surgical resection of the cardiac myxoma. Regarding management strategies, 33 patients (60%) were managed conservatively as the primary choice. In three cases (5.5%) there was chemotherapy treatment; in one case, radiotherapy. One patient was treated with stereotactic radiosurgery.

4. Discussion

Cardiac myxomas are the most common benign cardiac tumor in adults [58]. Myxoma cells most likely arise from resident pluripotent or multipotent mesenchymal stem cells, the embryonic remnants of which differentiate into endothelial cells, smooth muscle cells and other mesenchymal cells and this explains the most common occurrence of myxomas in the atrial septum [58,59]. Myxomas of the heart are most common in adults between the third and sixth decades of life. They can occur sporadically (more often in women) or be familial [1,2,58]. Familial occurrence has been shown to be associated with an autosomal dominant mutation of the PRKAR1A gene located on chromosome 17q2 [59,60]. Familial myxomas are usually multiple, recurrent and located outside the left atrium [61].

The genetic basis of intracranial aneurysms is very complex. In recent years, there has been a growing interest in the extracellular matrix surrounding cerebral vessels, as well as the role of matrix metalloproteinases [62,63]. Studies on the genetics of aneurysms have been aimed at elucidating causative genes or discovering new loci associated with aneurysm risk. Genome-wide association studies have used single nucleotide polymorphism data to discover several susceptibility loci, including the SOX17 and CDKN2A genes. The proteins encoded by these genes regulate endothelial function and blood vessel formation and so genetic variation that affects the extracellular matrix may have the greatest impact on the risk of aneurysms [62,64].

The clinical picture of CM includes symptoms due to embolism, intracardiac obstruction, size, location and mobility of the tumor [1,59]. Patients with small tumors may remain asymptomatic for years, or nonspecific symptoms may mimic systemic or cardiovascular disease [58].

Embolism associated with detachment of tumor fragments or thrombi occurs in 10–50% of patients with cardiac myxomas [59,65]. There has been no correlation between the risk of embolism and tumor size and some authors have suggested an association of such complications with chest trauma [66]. Most commonly, embolisms involve the cerebral arteries, where cavernous malformations and aneurysms can develop. Neurological complications are a very broad group of symptoms that include fainting and loss of consciousness, headache and dizziness, seizures, transient cerebral ischemia, stroke or rupture of aneurysms or vascular malformations [5,8,51]. Women in their fifth decade of life are most at risk for embolic stroke and acute embolic stroke may be the first manifestation of atrial myxoma in a young patient [58,59]. Sudden loss of consciousness after strenuous exercise is particularly important in the patient's history [58]. Embolism of the coronary artery is rare, and it is even believed that the coronary arteries are relatively resistant to embolism due to anatomical conditions [1,65,67]. Braun et al. [61] showed from their analysis that only 40 cases of myocardial infarction due to myxoma have been documented in the literature.

The etiology of myxomatous cerebral aneurysms is still unknown [40,59]. A few hypotheses have been put forward in terms of the pathogenesis of aneurysms. Based on the literature, two main theories can be identified. First, a neoplastic process theory proposes that myxoma cells adhere to and penetrate the endothelium, then grow in the subintimal layer and destroy the arterial wall. However, it should be remembered that the metastatic hypothesis does not imply a typical tumor metastasis process. By definition, cardiac myxomas are not malignant tumors and therefore do not have potential to "metastasize" in the strict sense of the word. The second theory is the "vascular damage theory" proposed by Sloane et al. in 1966, where the temporary occlusion of cerebral vessels by myxoma cells causes damage to the endothelium, which is followed by an alteration of hemodynamics and promotion of aneurysm formation [68–70].

Myxoma cells produce and release proinflammatory cytokine interleukin-6 (IL-6), which is an important factor of aneurysm initiation [18]. Recent studies suggest that autocrine production of IL-6 by myxoma plays a main role in the embolization of the myxomatous cell. Elevated IL-6 levels have been detected in patients with myxomatous aneurysms, before and even after myxoma resection. It has been known that atrial myxoma cells are capable of producing IL-6. Recent studies have shown that there is a connection between overproduction of Il-6 and cerebral aneurysm development. A persistent elevated IL-6 level induces overexpression of multiple proteolytic enzymes (such as metalloproteinase), which can weaken cerebral vessel walls and lead to aneurysm formation [55,71]. Based on this theory, cardiac myxoma resection is usually accompanied by a reduction in serum IL-6 levels, but a few studies have shown new aneurysm formation after the myxoma resection still showed persistently elevated IL-6 levels. Formation of a cerebral aneurysm is also associated with overproduction of Il-6 by an emboli tumor, that induces degradation of the extracellular matrix in the intracranial vessels and is connected with an increased level of IL-6 in cerebrospinal fluid. So, IL-6 has two ways of impacting the formation of the aneurysm's direction, first by promoting tumor invasion into the intracranial artery or secondly by increasing the chance of a distant embolization of the cardiac myxoma [55,57,71].

The natural history of this kind of aneurysm is also not clear; some cases have shown stability, others have shown improvement (self-occlusion) and others have shown an increased number and enlargement of aneurysms [5,51,57]. In most cases, the first neurological manifestation of atrial myxomas is complications due to cerebral embolism and subsequent cerebral infarction [2,59,65]. Vascular incidents (transient cerebral ischemia, stroke), which were observed in 36.3% of the patients of this review, should be precisely associated with embolism. Aneurysm formation and subsequent subarachnoid or intracerebral hemorrhage are rare but are the most well-known complications of atrial myxoma in adults [5]. Even the presence of multiple but unruptured cerebral vascular aneurysms usually does not produce clinical symptoms. However, up to half of patients with cerebral aneurysms may experience so-called "predictive headaches," the exact cause of which is not known, but is thought to be related to microbleeding from aneurysms or other vascular malformations [69,72,73]. The other symptoms that were observed in the patients analyzed in this review included seizures, headaches or dizziness that could be related to microbleeding from aneurysms or could be a symptom related to compression of malformations on central nervous system structures. Given some nonspecific but nevertheless quite suggestive clinical signs, it is necessary to screen for cerebral complications in patients with atrial myxoma.

Currently, there are no guidelines for the treatment of aneurysms caused by cardiac myxomas, but a conservative approach and radiological follow-up is recommended. The majority of reported cases have demonstrated stability and some have even been documented as exhibiting spontaneous regression [12]. Routine radiological follow-up by MRI examination is needed to monitor the eventual progression of the aneurysms [72,73]. A lot of therapeutic methods are available, ranging from endovascular methods, surgery, chemotherapy, radiation or a combination of these. Only enlarged or ruptured aneurysms may require invasive management and must be evaluated for endovascular or neurosurgical intervention [4].

The atrial myxoma should be excised as soon as possible after the diagnosis to prevent further complications such as systemic embolization, constitutional symptoms (fever, fatigue, weight loss) or obstruction of the mitral valve [44,58,59]. Surgical resection of the cardiac myxoma also eliminates the early neurologic symptoms, most frequently ischemic cerebral infarcts. Although the cardiac resection of the atrial tumor minimizes the risk of embolization, it does not decrease the risk of the formation of a delayed cerebral aneurysm. This results from the theory of "metastasis and infiltrate". Intracranial aneurysms may continue to grow despite the surgical removal of the atrial myxoma [53,67].

The current literature describes several different surgical options. Cases of ruptured aneurysms are generally considered as urgent surgical procedures. Clipping or coiling are not applicable for myxomatous aneurysms because they are multiple, located at distal vessels, fusiform and without a neck. The literature provides a few reports about clipping of large aneurysms [54]. Aneurysms might keep growing after endovascular coil embolization [31].

Open surgical treatment is recommended for a lesion-caused mass effect or in cases of single saccular aneurysms. A bypass is recommended for lesions with good collateral compensation and it is a reasonable option when sacrifice of the feeding artery may be required. Compared with other options, this procedure is technically challenging and is limited because it is difficult to apply in a variety of locations where aneurysms may occur [33].

Chemotherapy as a treatment was introduced by Roeltgen et al. in 1981 [74]. They tried doxorubicin in conjunction with surgery for recurrent atrial myxoma. In some cases, etoposide and carboplatin were also used [13,50]. Chemotherapy may protect patients against aneurysm growth [13]. Low-dose radiation in combination with chemotherapy has been reported as an effective method for degradation of metastasis [5,12,13]. A new option is frameless stereotactic radiosurgery (SRT), which is less invasive than endovascular or open surgery, avoids the systemic effects of chemotherapy, and limits toxicity to surrounding brain parenchyma compared to whole brain irradiation [5].

5. Conclusions

Cerebral aneurysms are rare complications of cardiac myxoma, which can appear many years after cardiologic treatment. They are twice as common in middle-aged women. The entire area of vascularization is most often located in the area of the middle cerebral artery. Vascular incidents, unspecific headaches and seizures are their most common clinical manifestations; their rupture and subarachnoid hemorrhages are relatively rare. We do not have any treatment guidelines as yet, however, in the case of myxoma aneurysms a long-term observation is recommended.

Therefore, long-term follow-up of patients with cardiac myxomas for possible co-occurrence of cerebral aneurysms and their complications is very important. In addition, patients with multiple cerebral aneurysms, especially those with a cardiac burden, should be alert to the possibility of cardiac myxoma.

Author Contributions: J.C.-Ł.—conceptualized and wrote the manuscript; S.B.—reviewed the manuscript; M.W.-P.—conceptualized, wrote and reviewed the manuscript. All authors have read and agreed to the published version of the manuscript.

Funding: Supported by Wroclaw Medical University.

Institutional Review Board Statement: The study was conducted according to the guidelines of The Declaration of Helsinki, and approved by the Ethics Committee of Wroclaw Medical University.

Informed Consent Statement: Not applicable.

Data Availability Statement: The data presented in this study are available upon request from the corresponding author. The data are not publicly available.

Conflicts of Interest: The authors declare no conflict of interest.

Abbreviations

ACA	anterior cerebral artery
CT	computed tomography
CTA	computed tomography angiography
DSA	digital subtraction angiography
ICA	internal carotid artery
MCA	middle cerebral artery
MRA	magnetic resonance angiography
MRI	magnetic resonance imaging
PCA	posterior cerebral artery
PICA	posterior inferior cerebellar artery
SWI	susceptibility weighted imaging

References

1. McManus, B. Primary tumors of the heart. In *Braunwald's Heart Disease, A Text Book of Cardiovascular Medicine*, 9th ed.; Mann, D.L., Douglas, P.Z., Libby, P., Bonow, R.O., Eds.; Elsevier Saunders: Philadelphia, PA, USA, 2012; pp. 1638–1650.
2. Aggarwal, S.K.; Barik, R.; Sarma, T.; Iyer, V.R.; Sai, V.; Mishra, J.; Voleti, C.D. Clinical presentation and investigation findings in cardiac myxomas: New insights from the developing world. *Am. Heart J.* **2007**, *154*, 1102–1107. [CrossRef] [PubMed]
3. Wan, Y.; Du, H.; Zhang, L.; Guo, S.; Xu, L.; Li, Y.; He, H.; Zhou, L.; Chen, Y.; Mao, L.; et al. Multiple cerebral metastases and metastatic aneurysms in patients with left atrial Myxoma: A case report. *BMC Neurol.* **2019**, *19*, 249. [CrossRef]
4. Samanidis, G.; Khoury, M.; Balanika, M.; Perrea, D.N. Current challenges in the diagnosis and treatment of cardiac myxoma. *Kardiol Pol.* **2020**, *78*, 269–277. [CrossRef] [PubMed]
5. Hau, M.; Poon, T.L.; Cheung, F.C. Neurological manifestations of atrial myxoma and stereotactic radiosurgery for metastatic aneurysms. *J. Radiosurg. SBRT* **2020**, *6*, 329–331. [PubMed]
6. Xie, X.; Li, X. Multiple cerebral aneurysms associated with cardiac myxoma. *J. Card Surg.* **2019**, *34*, 860–862. [CrossRef]
7. Moher, D.; Liberati, A.; Tetzlaff, J.; Altman, D.G.; PRISMA Group. Preferred reporting items for systematic reviews and meta-analyses: The PRISMA statement. *BMJ* **2009**, *339*, b2535. [CrossRef]
8. Alrohimi, A.; Putko, B.N.; Jeffery, D.; Van Dijk, R.; Chow, M.; McCombe, J.A. Cerebral Aneurysm in Association with Left Atrial Myxoma. *Can. J. Neurol. Sci.* **2019**, *46*, 637–639. [CrossRef]

9. Asranna, A.P.; Kesav, P.; Nagesh, C.; Sreedharan, S.E.; Kesavadas, C.; Sylaja, P.N. Cerebral aneurysms and metastases occurring as a delayed complication of resected atrial Myxoma: Imaging findings including high resolution Vessel Wall MRI. *Neuroradiology* **2017**, *59*, 427–429. [CrossRef]
10. Ashalatha, R.; Moosa, A.; Gupta, A.K.; Krishna Manohar, S.R.; Sandhyamani, S. Cerebral aneurysms in atrial myxoma: A delayed, rare manifestation. *Neurol. India* **2005**, *53*, 216–218. [CrossRef]
11. Baikoussis, N.G.; Siminelakis, S.N.; Kotsanti, A.; Achenbach, K.; Argyropoulou, M.; Goudevenos, J. Multiple cerebral mycotic aneurysms due to left atrial myxoma: Are there any pitfalls for the cardiac surgeon? *Hellenic J. Cardiol.* **2011**, *52*, 466–468.
12. Bernet, F.; Stulz, P.M.; Carrel, T.P. Long-term remission after resection, chemotherapy, and irradiation of a metastatic myxoma. *Ann. Thorac. Surg.* **1998**, *66*, 1791–1792. [CrossRef] [PubMed]
13. Branscheidt, M.; Frontzek, K.; Bozinov, O.; Valavanis, A.; Rushing, E.J.; Weller, M.; Wegener, S. Etoposide/carboplatin chemotherapy for the treatment of metastatic myxomatous cerebral aneurysms. *J. Neurol.* **2014**, *261*, 828–830. [CrossRef] [PubMed]
14. Chen, Z.; Wang, Y.L.; Ye, W.; Miao, Z.R.; Song, Q.B.; Ling, F. Multiple intracranial aneurysms as delayed complication of atrial myxoma. *Case Rep. Lit. Rev. Interv. Neuroradiol.* **2005**, *11*, 251–254.
15. Chow, D.H.; Chan, N.; Choy, C.; Chu, P.; Yuen, H.; Lau, C.; Lo, Y.; Tsui, P.; Mok, N. A lady with atrial myxoma presenting with myocardial infarction and cerebral aneurysm. *Int. J. Cardiol.* **2014**, *172*, e16–e18. [CrossRef] [PubMed]
16. Desousa, A.L.; Muller, J.; Campbell, R.; Batnitzky, S.; Rankin, L. Atrial myxoma: A review of the neurological complications, metastases, and recurrences. *J. Neurol. Neurosurg. Psychiatry* **1978**, *41*, 1119–1124. [CrossRef]
17. Eddleman, C.S.; Gottardi-Littell, N.R.; Bendok, B.R.; Batjer, H.H.; Bernstein, R.A. Rupture of cerebral myxomatous aneurysm months after resection of the primary cardiac tumor. *Neurocrit. Care* **2010**, *13*, 252–255. [CrossRef]
18. Ezerioha, N.; Feng, W. Intracardiac Myxoma, Cerebral aneurysms and elevated Interleukin-6. *Case Rep. Neurol.* **2015**, *7*, 152–155. [CrossRef]
19. Flores, P.L.; Haglund, F.; Bhogal, P.; Yeo Leong Litt, L.; Södermann, M. The dynamic natural history of cerebral aneurysms from cardiac myxomas: A review of the natural history of myxomatous aneurysms. *Interv. Neuroradiol.* **2018**, *24*, 277–283. [CrossRef]
20. Furuya, K.; Sasaki, T.; Yoshimoto, Y.; Okada, Y.; Fujimaki, T.; Kirino, T. Histologically verified cerebral aneurysm formation secondary to embolism from cardiac myxoma. *Case Rep. J. Neurosurg.* **1995**, *83*, 170–173. [CrossRef]
21. George, K.J.; Rennie, A.; Saxena, A. Multiple cerebral aneurysms secondary to cardiac myxoma. *Br. J. Neurosurg.* **2012**, *26*, 409–411. [CrossRef]
22. Gupta, M.M.; Agrawal, N. Oncotic cerebral aneurysms in a case of left atrial myxoma, role of imaging in diagnostics and treatment. *Pol. J. Radiol.* **2015**, *80*, 490–495. [CrossRef] [PubMed]
23. Herbst, M.; Wattjes, M.P.; Urbach, H.; Inhetvin-Hutter, C.; Becker, D.; Klockgether, T.; Hartmann, A. Cerebral embolism from left atrial myxoma leading to cerebral and retinal aneurysms: A case report. *AJNR Am. J. Neuroradiol.* **2005**, *26*, 666–669. [PubMed]
24. Iskandar, M.E.; Dimitrova, K.; Geller, C.M.; Hoffman, D.M.; Tranbaugh, R.F. Complicated sporadic cardiac myxomas: A second recurrence and myxomatous cerebral aneurysms in one patient. *Case Rep. Surg.* **2013**, *2013*, 642394. [CrossRef] [PubMed]
25. Ivanović, B.A.; Tadić, M.; Vraneš, M.; Orbović, B. Cerebral aneurysm associated with cardiac myxoma: Case report. *Bosn. J. Basic Med. Sci.* **2011**, *11*, 65–68. [CrossRef]
26. Jean, W.C.; Walski-Easton, S.M.; Nussbaum, E.S. Multiple intracranial aneurysms as delayed complications of an atrial myxoma: Case report. *Neurosurgery* **2001**, *49*, 200–203.
27. Josephson, S.A.; Johnston, S.C. Multiple stable fusiform intracranial aneurysms following atrial myxoma. *Neurology* **2005**, *64*, 526. [CrossRef]
28. Kim, H.; Park, E.-A.; Lee, W.; Chung, J.W.; Park, J.H. Multiple cerebral and coronary aneurysms in a patient with left atrial myxoma. *Int. J. Cardiovasc. Imaging* **2012**, *28*, 129–132. [CrossRef]
29. Koo, Y.-H.; Kim, T.-G.; Kim, O.-J.; Oh, S.-H. Multiple fusiform cerebral aneurysms and highly elevated serum interleukin-6 in cardiac myxoma. *J. Korean Neurosurg. Soc.* **2009**, *45*, 394–396. [CrossRef]
30. Krishnan, P.; Rajaraman, K.; Chowdhury, S.R.; Das, S. Multiple fusiform distal aneurysms in an operated case of atrial myxoma: Case report and review of literature. *Neurol. India* **2013**, *61*, 184–185. [CrossRef]
31. Lazarow, F.; Aktan, S.; Lanier, K.; Agola, J. Coil embolization of an enlarging fusiform myxomatous cerebral aneurysm. *Radiol. Case Rep.* **2018**, *13*, 490–494. [CrossRef]
32. Li, Q.; Shang, H.; Zhou, D.; Liu, R.; He, L.; Zheng, H. Repeated embolism and multiple aneurysms: Central nervous system manifestations of cardiac myxoma. *Eur. J. Neurol.* **2008**, *15*, 112–113. [CrossRef] [PubMed]
33. Namura, O.; Saitoh, M.; Moro, H.; Watanabe, H.; Sogawa, M.; Nishikura, K.; Hayashi, J.-I. A case of biatrial multiple myxomas with glandular structure. *Ann. Thorac. Cardiovasc. Surg.* **2007**, *13*, 423–427. [PubMed]
34. Oguz, K.K.; Firat, M.M.; Cila, A. Fusiform aneurysms detected 5 years after removal of an atrial myxoma. *Neuroradiology* **2001**, *43*, 990–992. [CrossRef] [PubMed]
35. Oomen, A.W.; Kuijpers, S.H. Cerebral aneurysms one year after resection of a cardiac myxoma. *Neth. Heart J.* **2013**, *21*, 307–309. [CrossRef] [PubMed]
36. Quan, K.; Song, J.; Zhu, W.; Chen, L.; Pan, Z.; Li, P.; Mao, Y. Repeated multiple intracranial hemorrhages induced by cardiac myxoma mimicking cavernous angiomas: A case report. *Chin. Neurosurg. J.* **2017**, *3*, 119–122. [CrossRef]
37. Penn, D.L.; Lanpher, A.B.; Klein, J.M.; Kozakewich, H.P.W.; Kahle, K.T.; Smith, E.R.; Orbach, D.B. Multimodal treatment approach in a patient with multiple intracranial myxomatous aneurysms. *J. Neurosurg. Pediatr.* **2018**, *21*, 315–321. [CrossRef] [PubMed]

38. Radoi, M.P.; Stefanescu, F.; Arsene, D. Brain metastases and multiple cerebral aneurysms from cardiac myxoma: Case report and review of the literature. *Br. J. Neurosurg.* **2012**, *26*, 893–895. [CrossRef] [PubMed]
39. Ryou, K.S.; Lee, S.-H.; Park, S.-H.; Park, J.; Hwang, S.-K.; Hamm, I.-S. Multiple fusiform myxomatous cerebral aneurysms in a patient with Carney complex. *J. Neurosurg.* **2008**, *109*, 318–320. [CrossRef] [PubMed]
40. Sabolek, M.; Bachus, R.; Arnold, G.; Storch, A.; Bachus-Banaschak, K. Multiple cerebral aneurysms as delayed complication of left cardiac myxoma: A case report and review. *Acta Neurol. Scand.* **2005**, *111*, 345–350. [CrossRef]
41. Saffie, P.; Riquelme, F.; Mura, J.; Urra, A.; Passig, C.; Castro, Á.; Illanes, S. Multiple myxomatous aneurysms with bypass and clipping in a 37-year-old man. *J. Stroke Cerebrovasc. Dis.* **2015**, *24*, e69–e71. [CrossRef]
42. Santillan, A.; Sigounas, D.; Fink, M.E.; Gobin, Y.P. Multiple fusiform intracranial aneurysms 14 years after atrial myxoma resection. *Arch. Neurol.* **2012**, *69*, 1204–1205. [CrossRef]
43. Sato, T.; Saji, N.; Kobayashi, K.; Shibazaki, K.; Kimura, K. A case of cerebral embolism due to cardiac myxoma presenting with multiple cerebral microaneurysms detected on first MRI scans. *Rinsho Shinkeigaku* **2016**, *56*, 98–103. [CrossRef] [PubMed]
44. Sedat, J.; Chau, Y.; Dunac, A.; Gomez, N.; Suissa, L.; Mahagne, M. Multiple cerebral aneurysms caused by cardiac myxoma. A case report and present state of knowledge. *Interv. Neuroradiol.* **2007**, *13*, 179–184. [CrossRef] [PubMed]
45. Sorenson, T.J.; Brinjikji, W.; Lanzino, G. Giant Fusiform Intracranial Aneurysm in Patient with History of Myxoma. *World Neurosurg.* **2019**, *128*, 200–201. [CrossRef] [PubMed]
46. Srivastava, S.; Tewari, P. Stroke associated with left atrial mass: Association of cerebral aneurysm with left atrial myxoma. *Ann. Card. Anaesth.* **2014**, *17*, 56–58.
47. Stock, K. Multiple cerebral aneurysms in a patient with recurrent cardiac myxomas. A case report. *Interv. Neuroradiol.* **2004**, *10*, 335–340. [CrossRef]
48. Sveinsson, O.; Herrman, L. Multiple cerebral aneurysms in a patient with cardiac myxoma: What to do? *BMJ Case Rep.* **2015**, *2015*, bcr2013200767. [CrossRef]
49. Tamulevičiūtė, E.; Taeshineetanakul, P.; Terbrugge, K.; Krings, T. Myxomatous aneurysms: A case report and literature review. *Interv. Neuroradiol.* **2011**, *17*, 188–194. [CrossRef]
50. Vontobel, J.; Huellner, M.; Stolzmann, P. Cerebral 'metastasizing' cardiac myxoma. *Eur. Heart J.* **2016**, *37*, 1680. [CrossRef]
51. Waliszewska-Prosół, M.; Zimny, A.; Chojdak-Łukasiewicz, J.; Zagrajek, M.; Paradowski, B. Multiple fusiform cerebral aneurysms detected after atrial myxoma resection: A report of two cases. *Kardiol. Pol.* **2018**, *76*, 1571. [CrossRef]
52. Walker, M.; Kilani, R.; Toye, L.R. Central and peripheral fusiform aneurysms six years after left atrial myxoma resection. *J Neurol. Neurosurg. Psychiatry* **2003**, *74*, 277–282. [CrossRef]
53. Xu, Q.; Zhang, X.; Wu, P.; Wang, M.; Zhou, Y.; Feng, Y. Multiple intracranial aneurysms followed left atrial myxoma: Case report and literature review. *J. Thorac. Dis.* **2013**, *5*, E227–E231.
54. Yilmaz, M.B.; Akin, Y.; Güray, Ü.; Kisacik, H.L.; Korkmaz, S. Late recurrence of left atrial myxoma with multiple intracranial aneurysms. *Int. J. Cardiol.* **2003**, *87*, 303–305. [CrossRef] [PubMed]
55. Yokomuro, H.; Yoshihara, K.; Watanabe, Y.; Shiono, N.; Koyama, N.; Takanashi, Y. The variations in the immunologic features and interleukin-6 levels for the surgical treatment of cardiac myxomas. *Surg. Today* **2007**, *37*, 750–753. [CrossRef]
56. Zeng, T.; Ji, Z.Y.; Shi, S.S. Atrial myxoma presenting with multiple intracranial fusiform aneurysms: A case report. *Acta Neurol. Belg.* **2015**, *115*, 453–455. [CrossRef]
57. Zhang, R.; Tang, Z.; Qiao, Q.; Mahmood, F.; Feng, Y. Anesthesia management of atrial myxoma resection with multiple cerebral aneurysms: A case report and review of the literature. *BMC Anesthesiol.* **2020**, *20*, 164. [CrossRef] [PubMed]
58. Jaravaza, D.R.; Lalla, U.; Zaharie, S.D.; de Jager, L.J. Unusual Presentation of Atrial Myxoma: A Case Report and Review of the Literature. *Am. J. Case Rep.* **2021**, *22*, e931437. [CrossRef] [PubMed]
59. Reynen, K. Cardiac myxomas. *N. Engl. J. Med.* **1995**, *333*, 1610–1617. [CrossRef] [PubMed]
60. Wen, X.; Chen, Y.; Yu, L.; Wang, S.; Zheng, H.; Chen, Z.; Ma, L.; Liao, X.; Li, Q. Neurological manifestations of atrial myxoma: A retrospective analysis. *Oncol. Lett.* **2018**, *16*, 4635–4639. [CrossRef]
61. Braun, S.; Schrötter, H.; Reynen, K.; Schwencke, C.; Strasser, R.H. Myocardial infarction as complication of left atrial myxoma. *Int. J. Cardiol.* **2005**, *101*, 115–121. [CrossRef]
62. Dagra, A.; Williams, E.; Aghili-Mehrizi, S.; Goutnik, M.A.; Martinez, M.; Turner, R.C.; Lucke-Wold, B. Pediatric Subarachnoid Hemorrhage: Rare Events with Important Implications. *Brain Neurol. Disord.* **2022**, *5*, 020. [CrossRef] [PubMed]
63. Laurent, D.; Small, C.; Lucke-Wold, B.; Dodd, W.S.; Chalouhi, N.; Hu, Y.C.; Hosaka, K.; Motwani, K.; Martinez, M.; Polifka, A.; et al. Understanding the genetics of intracranial aneurysms: A primer. *Clin. Neurol. Neurosurg.* **2022**, *212*, 107060. [CrossRef] [PubMed]
64. Foroud, T.; Koller, D.L.; Lai, D.; Sauerbeck, L.; Anderson, C.; Ko, N.; Deka, R.; Mosley, T.H.; Fornage, M.; Woo, D.; et al. FIA Study Investigators. Genome-wide association study of intracranial aneurysms confirms role of Anril and SOX17 in disease risk. *Stroke* **2012**, *43*, 2846–2852. [CrossRef] [PubMed]
65. Waikar, H.D.; Jayakrishnan, A.G.; Bandusena, B.S.N.; Priyadarshan, P.; Kamalaneson, P.P.; Ileperuma, A.; Neema, P.K.; Dhawan, R.; Chaney, M.A. Left atrial myxoma presenting as cerebral embolism. *J. Cardiothorac. Vasc. Anesth.* **2020**, *34*, 3452–3461. [CrossRef]
66. Cho, W.C.; Trivedi, A. Widespread systemic and peripheral embolization of left atrial myxoma following blunt chest trauma. *Conn. Med.* **2017**, *81*, 153–156.
67. Al Zahrani, I.M.; Alraqtan, A.; Rezk, A.; Almasswary, A.; Bella, A. Atrial myxoma related myocardial infarction: Case report and review of the literature. *J. Saudi Heart Assoc.* **2014**, *26*, 166–169. [CrossRef]

68. Sloane, L.; Allen, J.H.; Collins, H.A. Radiologic observations in cerebral embolization from left heart myxoma. *Radiology* **1966**, *87*, 262e6.
69. Lee, V.H.; Connolly, H.M.; Brown, R.D., Jr. Central nervous system manifestations of cardiac myxoma. *Arch. Neurol.* **2007**, *64*, 1115–1120. [CrossRef]
70. Pinede, L.; Duhaut, P.; Loire, R. Clinical presentation of left atrial cardiac myxoma. A series of 112 consecutive cases. *Medicine* **2001**, *80*, 159–172. [CrossRef]
71. Mendoza, C.E.; Rosado, M.F.; Bernal, L. The role of interleukin-6 in cases of cardiac myxoma. Clinical features, immunologic abnormalities, and a possible role in recurrence. *Tex. Heart. Inst. J.* **2001**, *28*, 3–7.
72. Nucifora, P.G.; Dillon, W.P. MRI diagnosis of myxomatous aneurysms: Report of two cases. *AJNR Am. J. Neuroradiol.* **2001**, *22*, 1349–1352. [PubMed]
73. Chiang, K.-H.; Cheng, H.-M.; Chang, B.-S.; Chiu, C.-H.; Yen, P.-S. Multiple cerebral aneurysms as manifestations of cardiac myxoma: Brain imaging, digital subtraction angiography, and echocardiography. *Tzu Chi Med. J.* **2011**, *23*, 63–65. [CrossRef]
74. Roeltgen, D.P.; Weimer, G.R.; Patterson, L.F. Delayed neurologic complications of left atrial myxoma. *Neurology* **1981**, *31*, 8–13. [CrossRef] [PubMed]

Disclaimer/Publisher's Note: The statements, opinions and data contained in all publications are solely those of the individual author(s) and contributor(s) and not of MDPI and/or the editor(s). MDPI and/or the editor(s) disclaim responsibility for any injury to people or property resulting from any ideas, methods, instructions or products referred to in the content.

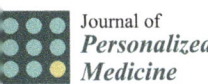

Article

Minimally Invasive Isolated and Hybrid Surgical Revascularization for Multivessel Coronary Disease: A Single-Center Long-Term Follow-Up

Tiziano Torre [1,†], Alberto Pozzoli [1,*,†], Marco Valgimigli [2,3], Laura Anna Leo [2], Francesca Toto [1], Mirko Muretti [1], Sara Birova [1], Enrico Ferrari [1,3,4], Giovanni Pedrazzini [2,3] and Stefanos Demertzis [1,3,5]

1 Heart Surgery Unit, Cardiocentro Ticino Institute, EOC, 6900 Lugano, Switzerland; tiziano.torre@eoc.ch (T.T.); francesca.toto@eoc.ch (F.T.); mirko.muretti@eoc.ch (M.M.); sara.birova@eoc.ch (S.B.); enrico.ferrari@eoc.ch (E.F.); stefanos.demertzis@eoc.ch (S.D.)
2 Cardiology Unit, Cardiocentro Ticino Institute, EOC, 6900 Lugano, Switzerland; lauraanna.leo@eoc.ch (L.A.L.); giovanni.pedrazzini@eoc.ch (G.P.)
3 Faculty of Biomedical Sciences, Università della Svizzera Italiana (USI), 6900 Lugano, Switzerland
4 Faculty of Medicine, University of Zurich (UZH), 8032 Zurich, Switzerland
5 Faculty of Medicine, University of Bern, 3010 Bern, Switzerland
* Correspondence: alberto.pozzoli@eoc.ch
† These authors contributed equally to this work.

Abstract: Introduction: Some evidence suggests that surgical minimally invasive (MIDCAB) and hybrid coronary revascularization (HCR) are safe and potentially effective at short-term follow-up. Data on long-term outcomes are more limited and inconclusive. Methods: Between February 2013 and December 2023, a total of 1997 patients underwent surgical coronary artery revascularization at our institution, of whom, 92 (4.7%) received left anterior mini-thoracotomy access (MIDCAB), either isolated (N = 78) or in combination with percutaneous coronary intervention (N = 14, HCR group). Results: After a median follow-up of 75 months (range 3.1: 149 months), cardiac mortality was 0% while overall mortality was 3%, with one in-hospital mortality and two additional late deaths. Conversion to sternotomy happened in two patients (2.1%), and surgical re-explorations occurred in five patients (4.6%), of whom three for bleeding and two for graft failure. All patients received left internal mammary (LIMA) to left anterior descending artery (LAD) grafting (100%). In the HCR group, 10 patients (72%) showed percutaneous revascularization (PCI) after MIDCAB, showing PCI on a mean of 1.6 ± 0.6 vessels and implanting 2.1 ± 0.9 drug-eluting stents. Conclusions: MIDCAB, in isolation or in association with hybrid coronary revascularization, is associated with encouraging short- and long-term results in selected patients discussed within a dedicated heart-team.

Keywords: multivessel coronary disease; minimally invasive coronary bypass surgery; MIDCAB; beating-heart coronary surgery; hybrid coronary revascularization; percutaneous coronary intervention; heart team

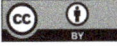

1. Introduction

Coronary artery bypass grafting (CABG) is the most common adult surgery procedure performed globally as well as the foundation of cardiac surgery, which has evolved considerably since the time of its introduction approximately 50 years ago [1].

Minimally invasive direct coronary artery bypass (MIDCAB) grafting has been suggested as an effective and less invasive alternative to traditional CABG for the revascularization of the left anterior descending artery [2,3]. Over the last twenty years, the aim to achieve more extensive revascularization, maintaining a minimally invasive approach, has led many experienced surgeons to treat multivessel disease, too [4]. The results of the Syntax (Synergy Between Percutaneous Coronary Intervention with Taxus and Cardiac Surgery) Trial in 2014 clearly showed that surgery is the gold standard for three-vessel coronary disease, especially for those individuals with complex anatomies. Surgical revascularization was shown to be superior to percutaneous coronary intervention (PCI) with a first-generation drug-eluting stent (DES) with respect to the composite endpoint of death, myocardial infarction, stroke, and repeated revascularization [5]. On the other hand, a high rate of saphenous vein graft failures, sternal complications, and bleeding events have been observed in CABG patients. The routine use of second-generation DES was subsequently shown to be associated with a lower rate of restenosis and thrombosis than saphenous graft failure [6–8]. These results led, in 2018, to a statement of the European guidelines for CABG to be the standard treatment for multivessel disease (Figure 1), when a left internal mammary artery (LIMA) to left anterior descending (LAD) grafting is performed. Since the new generation DES provides satisfactory short- and long-term clinical outcomes, the armamentarium would be considered high quality on both arms [7]. In fact, saphenous vein grafts (SVG) exhibit lower patency and a higher mortality rate compared with those of LIMA. The SVGs have been shown to occlude (up to 50%) as early as 10 years after implantation due to many factors [8]. The failure of these grafts reached a rate of 30% to 40% after 10 years, due to patients developing SVG intimal hyperplasia. In addition to intimal thickening, SVGs can undergo atherosclerosis, with angiographic studies demonstrating an attrition rate of the SVG of 2% from the first to the seventh post-operative year with only 38% to 45% of SVGs remaining patent after 10 years [8]. Hence, the introduction in clinical practice of a hybrid coronary revascularization (HCR) to deal with multivessel coronary artery disease has been based on the wish to combine the best of the two therapies (Figures 2 and 3). In 2011, the Guidelines of the American College of Cardiology (ACC) recommended a Class II a for hybrid revascularization, indicated only in selected patients not otherwise approachable with traditional surgical or percutaneous revascularization [9]. However, there are only a few randomized trials in the literature supporting the evidence, one of which was prematurely discontinued for suboptimal enrollment, which led to inconclusive recommendations from the most recent Guidelines [10]. Due to the lack of robust evidence supporting the HCR strategy, our daily clinical practice could only be based on the studies comparing HCR to traditional CABG or PCI. The aim of this original article is to report the outcomes of our institutional program on isolated and hybrid minimally invasive coronary surgery. Furthermore, the strategies adopted within the Heart Team according to the Guidelines will be discussed, with respect to the indication, timing, and staging of the two procedures.

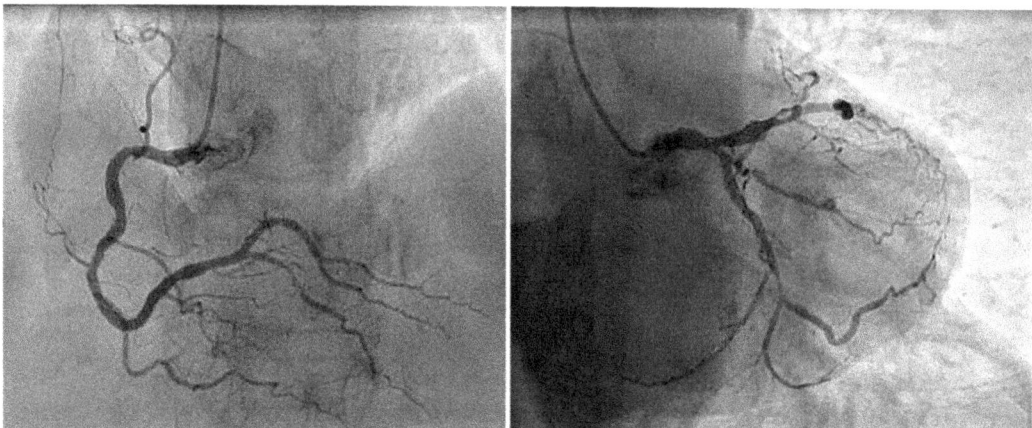

Figure 1. Preoperative coronary angiogram of an 80-year-old patient suffering from multivessel coronary disease on the distal right coronary artery (**left**) and diffusely on the left coronary system (**right**).

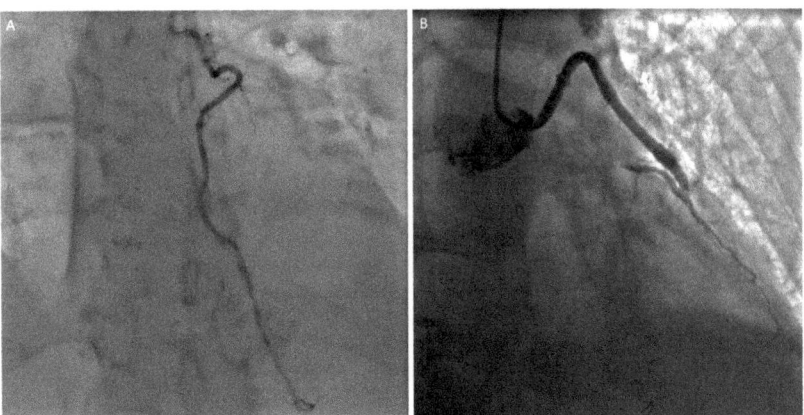

Figure 2. Postoperative coronary angiogram after bypass surgery performed in a minimally invasive fashion on the left anterior descending (LAD) with the left internal mammary artery (LIMA) (**A**) and the angiographic result of the venous graft on the diagonal branch (**B**).

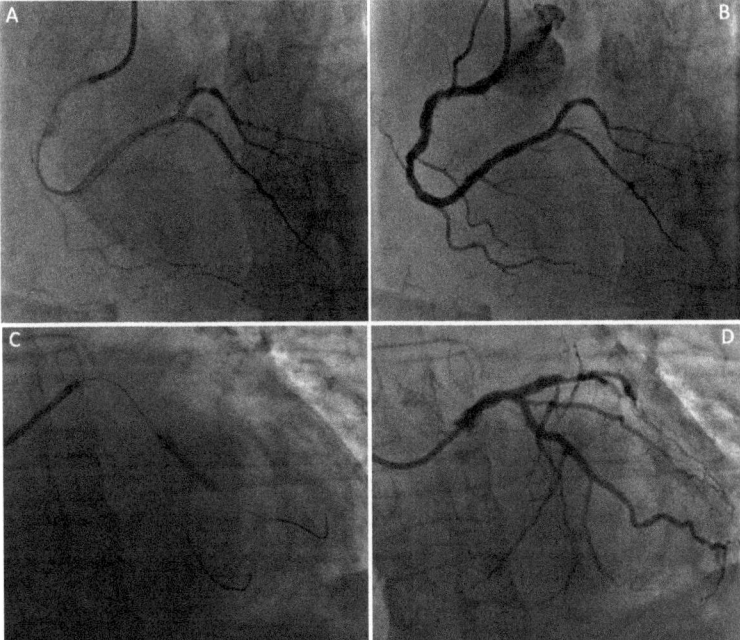

Figure 3. Four panel figure depicting the PCI treatment with stenting of the non-LAD vessels. Panel (**A**,**B**): angiographic result after percutaneous revascularization (PCI) with a drug-eluting stent on the distal portion of the right coronary artery. Panel (**C**,**D**): angiographic result after percutaneous revascularization (PCI) with a drug-eluting stent at the obtuse marginals' bifurcation of the circumflex coronary artery.

2. Materials and Methods

2.1. Study Design

Between February 2013 and December 2023, a total of 1997 patients with coronary artery disease were referred for CABG at our Institution. Within this study period, MIDCAB and HCR patients were extracted. Baseline patient characteristics and surgical details were prospectively collected in the institutional electronic medical database and retrospectively analyzed for this study. The study was conducted according to the privacy policy of the Cardiocentro Ticino Institute and the internal regulations for the appropriate use of anonymized data in patient-oriented research, which are based on international regulations, including the Declaration of Helsinki (MEC-2020-0454). All patients signed informed consent forms for surgery and the Ethics Committee of Canton of Ticino approved the study design (CE 3103/BASEC 2016-0519, approval date: 22 March 2017). The follow-up was conducted either by analyzing the hospital medical records or via telephone calls to the patients or the general practitioners. In case of no response, we questioned the national mortuary office. The follow-up ended in December 2023.

2.2. Inclusion and Exclusion Criteria for MIDCAB /HCR and Pharmacologic Strategy

All patients were discussed within the Heart Team, either for isolated MIDCAB surgery or MIDCAB combined with percutaneous treatment of non-LAD vessels for a hybrid revascularization strategy, according to the international Guidelines [10].

To perform MIDCAB surgery at our institution, a combination of multiple inclusion criteria was mandatory, divided into three different domains, namely, anatomical, physiological, and surgical:

- Favorable chest anatomy to properly expose the heart and absence of calcifications or obstructing plaques of the femoral arteries, in case a peripheral cannulation for the cardiopulmonary bypass, would be needed.
- Hemodynamic stability and an adequate pulmonary function to tolerate single lung ventilation.
- Absence of calcification of the ascending aorta, allowing the execution of the proximal anastomosis (Figure 4A).

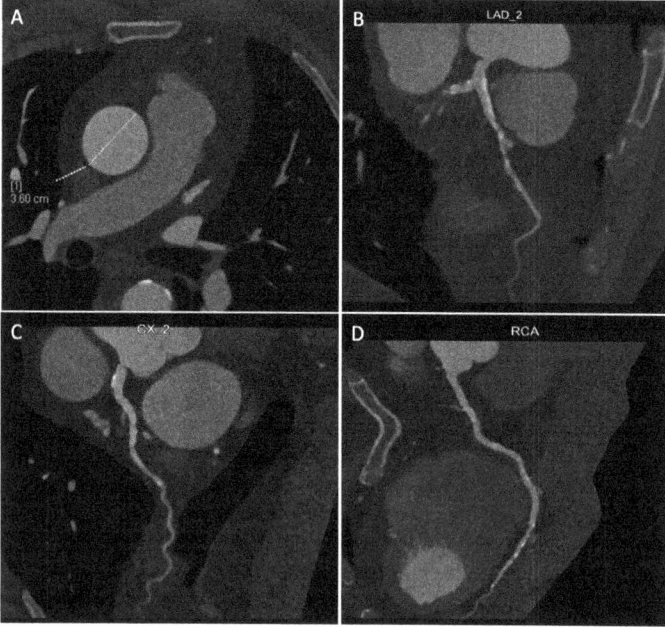

Figure 4. Coronary multislice computed tomography (MSCT) performed before the operation, with the analysis of the ascending aorta (**A**) and of the three epicardial coronaries (**B–D**), including the left main. [1] It refers to the calculated diameter of the ascending aorta (white dashed and solid lines).

Absolute contraindications to MIDCAB at our institution are severe chest wall deformities (e.g., pectus excavatum), severe lung pathologies, and, obviously, emergent surgery with hemodynamic instability.

The MIDCAB was preferentially performed as a first-stage procedure within an HCR strategy and followed by PCI on the other vessels whenever feasible. Instead, culprit lesions were treated percutaneously during the same hospitalization or, if clinically feasible, in a new hospitalization at least one month after discharge. One hundred milligrams of acetylsalicylic acid was administered before the operation and continued indefinitely. The antiplatelet regimen included a loading dose of clopidogrel 300 mg or ticagrelor 180 mg at the time of PCI, with a recommended treatment duration of 12 months.

In patients with acute coronary syndrome, the culprit lesion on the non-LAD vessel is treated immediately and the surgical revascularization on the LAD is staged thereafter. Other non-LAD vessels were scheduled based on the severity of the lesions. In these patients, the P2Y12 receptor inhibitor was discontinued 3 to 5 days before the admission and/or surgery, and intravenous Cangrelor was used to embricate the P2Y12 receptor inhibitor. Every case is evaluated by the Multiplate® Analyzer (Roche, Rotkreuz, Switzerland) to test the platelet function and confirm the operability. The DAPT therapy was to be reintroduced on the second postoperative day and continued according to individual bleeding and ischemic risks.

2.3. Preoperative Planning

All patients undergoing MIDCAB intervention, beyond coronary angiogram and a baseline transthoracic echocardiography, require further imaging with a cardiac multislice computed tomography (MSCT) with 3D reconstruction of the target vessels (left anterior descending artery particularly, then the diagonal or lateral/posterolateral branches) to exclude an intra-myocardial course, identify the target zone for the coronary anastomosis, and analyze the ascending aorta (Figures 4A–D and 5).

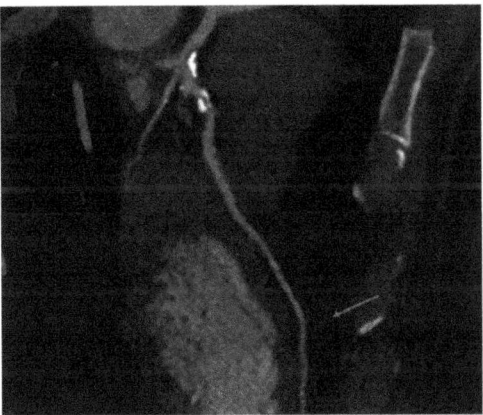

Figure 5. The coronary multislice computed tomography (MSCT), depicting—red arrow—the intramyocardial course of the left anterior descending (LAD), which represents a fundamental exclusion criteria prior to minimally invasive coronary surgery (MIDCAB).

2.4. Surgical Technique

All patients were positioned in a semi-supine position and the left chest was elevated at 30°. General mixed anesthesia was induced. An invasive arterial blood pressure monitoring (preferably right radial artery) was obtained. The intubation was performed with the use of a double-lumen endotracheal tube. A central venous port was introduced through the right jugular vein. A Foley catheter was passed into the bladder. Transesophageal echocardiography (TEE) was adopted in every patient. The groins were prepared in case of hemodynamic instability needing cardiopulmonary bypass. A left anterolateral mini-thoracotomy of 5 to 7 cm was performed in the sub-mammary crease according to the particular case. Since 2020, depending on the incision and procedure, a combination of intercostal, pectoralis, and serratus anterior nerve blockades have been adopted. The skin in the crease was marked the day before the operation, with the patient carefully seated on the bed and the pectoral muscles relaxed. In the operating room, the left internal mammary artery (LIMA) was harvested in a skeletonized fashion and under direct vision through the fourth intercostal space. At the beginning of our experience in 2013, we adopted the MIDAccess IMA retractor system (Delacroix-Chevalier, Paris, France) and starting in 2019, the MICS CABG Fehling retractor (Fehling Instruments, Karlstein am Main, Germany), which allowed either the left and the right internal thoracic artery harvesting. After opening and suspending the pericardium in a circular fashion, the left anterior descending (LAD) was identified, along with its target point of anastomosis, to check the effective length of the grafts. Heparin was administered in a standard dose of 10.000 UI to achieve an activated clotting time > 250 s. A disposable suction Medtronic Octopus stabilizer (Medtronic Inc., Minneapolis, MI, USA) was routinely adopted. In case of difficult exposure of the targeted vessels, including the lateral and inferior walls, a transthoracic stabilizer was favored (Nuvo, Medtronic Inc., Minneapolis, MI, USA). For the distal anastomosis, once the epicardium was stabilized, a blower was adopted to visualize the anastomotic area, and an intracoronary shunt was always inserted into the artery. The anastomotic suture was usually executed with a polypropylene 8-0 monofilament, with standard coronary instruments. In case proximal anastomosis or aortic cross-clamping were required, the ascending aorta was encircled with a Dacron tape, in order to freely mobilize it and enhance the exposure. In the case of hemodynamic instability or in the case of suboptimal target vessel exposure, the cardiopulmonary bypass could be instituted via peripheral femoral vessels. Every coronary conduit was assessed with a flow probe based on TransitTime Flow Measurement (TTFM) by Medistim ASA (Oslo, Norway) at the end. At chest closure, one Blake 24 Fr soft drain was routinely placed in the left pleural space via the 6th intercostal incision. Usually, the left lung has been gently re-inflated to avoid damage to the graft(s). The two ribs were normally tied together with a 2-0 Vicryl-coated suture. The skin closure was performed with 4-0 STRATAFIX™ Spiral Knotless (Figure 6). Postoperative analgesia was enhanced by slow a continuous anesthetic delivery of bupivacaine of 5% through small catheters positioned inside the wound.

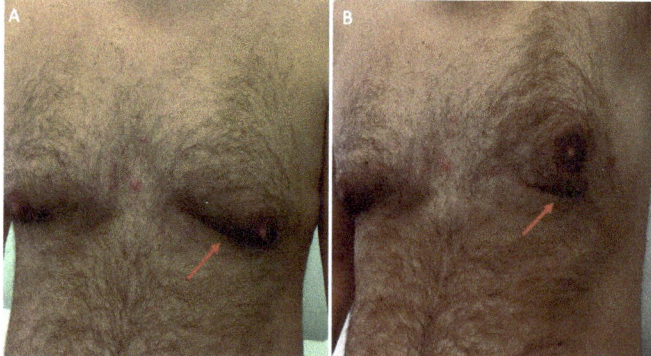

Figure 6. Postoperative cosmetic result after minimally invasive bypass surgery, implanting the left internal mammary artery on the left anterior descending. The reduced scar is visible (red arrows) in the submammary crease with the left arm at rest (**A**) and with the left arm raised (**B**).

2.5. Statistical Analysis

The statistical analysis was performed using Stata 17 (StataCorp, College Station, TX, USA). Continuous variables are presented as mean ± standard deviation and categorical variables are presented as numbers and percentages.

3. Results

Between February 2013 and December 2023, a total of 1997 patients with coronary artery disease were referred for CABG at our institution. Ninety-two of them (4.6%) were operated on through a left anterior mini-thoracotomy access. In the period from January 2017 to November 2023, 14 patients out of 92 (15%) underwent a hybrid revascularization strategy. Demographic and clinical characteristics of both groups are reported in detail below (Table 1). The intraoperative data are listed in Table 2. After a median follow-up of 75 months (range 3.1:149 months), cardiac mortality was 0% and overall mortality was 3%, with one case of in-hospital mortality (1%), a patient who developed a subarachnoid hemorrhage on the 5th postoperative day, and two additional late deaths. When the conversion rate to sternotomy was analyzed, two cases converted due to the intramyocardial course of the LAD were detected (2.1%). Surgical re-explorations were needed in three patients for bleeding (No bleeding was caused by having the double antiplatelets therapy (DAPT), either in patients receiving single surgical coronary bypass (isolated group) or in patients treated with a hybrid approach (hybrid group) and in two cases for revision due to graft failure (4.6%). Postoperative complications for the total MIDCAB and for the hybrid group are reported in Table 3. All patients received a LIMA to LAD grafting, and in 22 cases (24.2%), one more graft was executed. In the hybrid group, the LIMA has been used as a single graft on the LAD for every patient (Figure 2A), while in two of them, it has also been grafted to the first diagonal branch (Figure 2B). Seventy-nine patients were extubated directly in the operative room (86%) and all patients in the HCR group were extubated directly at the end of surgery (Table 3). Patients in the hybrid group underwent a two-staged PCI revascularizing a mean of 1.6 ± 0.6 vessels (Table 4). In five patients, the procedure was performed during the same hospitalization, while in another three patients, the procedure was scheduled beyond 30 days following the indexed revascularization. The follow-up was conducted until December 2023, and it was 95% complete. The mortality data rate during the follow-up was 100% complete and based on the consultation of the Swiss death bulletin (https://www.todesanzeigenportal.ch, accessed on 1 February 2024).

Table 1. Demographic and clinical characteristics.

	N (Percentage %)	
	Tot. MIDCAB	Hybrid
Patients	92 (100%)	14/92 (1.5%)
Age (years)	67.9 ± 10.4	72 ± 10.5
Male	81 (88%)	12 (86%)
Smoking	23 (25%)	4 (29%)
Hypertension	64 (70%)	13 (93%)
Dyslipidemia	61 (66%)	9 (64%)
Chronic coronary syndrome	25 (27%)	2 (14%)
Unstable angina	67 (73%)	12 (86%)
History of myocardial infarction	26 (28%)	2 (14%)
Diabetes type I under insulin therapy	13 (14%)	1 (7%)
Diabetes type II	28 (30%)	4 (29%)
PAD	7 (8%)	0 (0%)
Number of diseased vessels (N, %)	1 vessel: 33 (36%) 2 vessels: 47 (51%) 3 vessels: 12 (13%)	1 vessel: 0 (0%) 2 vessels: 9 (64%) 3 vessels: 5 (36%)
Euroscore II	1.0 ± 0.7	0.95 ± 0.5
Ejection Fraction (%)	56 ± 7.5	53 ± 6.2

Data are expressed as mean value ± standard deviation (SD). PAD: Peripheral Artery Disease.

Table 2. Intraoperative data.

		N (Percentage %)	
		Tot. MIDCAB	Hybrid
N° of bypass			
	1	58 (63%)	12 (86%)
	2	30 (33%)	2 (14%)
	3	4 (4%)	0 (0%)
Lima		92 (100%)	14 (100%)
	+ Rima	4 (4%)	0 (0%)
	+ Radial	1 (1%)	0 (0%)
	+ SVG	17 (18%)	0 (0%)
Op. time (min)		210 ± 85	178 ± 65
CPB time in 7 cases (min)		117 ± 41	0 (0%)
X-Clamp time in 2 cases (min)		62	0 (0%)

Data are expressed as mean value ± standard deviation (SD). Lima: Left Internal Mammary Artery; Rima: Right Internal Mammary Artery; SVG: Saphenous Vein Graft; CPB: Cardiopulmonary Bypass.

Table 3. Postoperative Complications.

		N (Percentage %)	
		Tot. MIDCAB	Hybrid
30-day Mortality		1 (1%)	0
Extubation			
	POD 0	79 (86%)	14 (100%)
	POD 1	11 (12%)	0 (0%)
	POD > 1	2 (2%)	0 (0%)
Graft failure		2 (2.1)	0 (0%)
Sternotomy conversion		2 (2.1)	0 (0%)
Surgical revision		3 (3.2)	0 (0%)
ICU stay (days)		1.3 ± 0.7	1
Post-operative Hospital stay (days)		6.4 ± 3.9	6.3 ± 1.3
Long-term Mortality		2 (2.1%)	0 (0%)

Data are expressed as mean value ± standard deviation (SD). POD: Post-Operative Day; ICU: Intensive Care Unit.

Table 4. Hybrid coronary revascularization strategy.

	Hybrid Coronary Revascularization (14 Patients)
N° of treated vessels (out of LAD)	1.6 ± 0.6
N° of treated vessels (out of LAD) per patient (N, %)	
- 1 vessel	6/14 (43%)
- 2 vessels	7/14 (50%)
- 3 vessels	1/14 (7%)
N° of Drug Eluting Stent (mean ± SD)	2.1 ± 0.9
Type of Drug Eluting Stent (target vessels)	ORSIRO (RCA) BIOFREEDOM (RCA) XIENCE SIERRA (RCA and CX) ULTIMASTER TANSEI (RCA and CX) ORSIRO MISSION (RCA and RCX) XIENCE SKYPOINT (RCA) RESOLUTE ONYX (PDA) ONYX FRONTIER (RCA and PLA) ULTIMASTER NAGOMI (RI)
PCI before Surgery (n° of pts, %)	4 (28%)

Table 4. Cont.

	Hybrid Coronary Revascularization (14 Patients)
Days before Surgery (mean ± SD)	28 ± 21
PCI after Surgery (n° of pts, %)	10 (72%)
Days after Surgery (mean ± SD)	31 ± 24
LIMA angiographic patency at staged PCI (n° of pts, %)	10 (100%)
PCI during the same hospitalization (n° of pts, %)	5 (36%)
Re-exploration for bleeding due to DAPT	0 (0%)

LAD: left anterior descending; PCI: percutaneous coronary revascularization; DAPT: dual antiplatelet therapy; SD: standard deviation; RCA: right coronary artery; PDA: posterior descending artery; CX: circumflex artery; PLA: posterolateral artery; RI: ramus intermedius.

4. Discussion

Minimally invasive coronary artery bypass represents an interesting and valid option for surgical myocardial revascularization in selected patients.

This work conveys at least three relevant messages regarding minimally invasive and hybrid revascularization strategies:

a. One of the main advantages results from the avoidance of sternotomy, hence the risk for sternal wound infections (or mediastinitis) and sternal instability are completely abolished.
b. For solely surgical revascularization of the LAD by a left mini-thoracotomy, followed by staged PCI, our results demonstrate that the long-term patency rate is as good as with sternotomy.
c. Although only in a limited number of patients, the management of DAPT demonstrated a good safety profile and low bleeding risk in those patients in whom MIDCAB has been staged after PCI.

Having said that, if the association between surgery and percutaneous revascularization is adopted to achieve complete revascularization in multivessel disease, the hybrid strategy can be considered a viable one. The key question relates to the right patient selection, for whom the isolated minimally invasive or the hybrid revascularization strategy should be performed. Revising the existing literature and relative outcomes would help to answer this clinical question. One of the first large studies on MIDCAB, analyzing 300 patients, documented a short-term LIMA patency of 98% and a repeat revascularization rate of 4% [11]. In a meta-analysis by Raja et al. on about eight thousand patients, the results of LAD treatment comparing MIDCAB and PCI showed no differences in mortality, myocardial infarctions, and MACCE rate, with MIDCAB reporting a superior freedom from repeat revascularization [12]. One of the first prospective randomized trials published in 2018, the POL-MIDES Trial, compared the results of hybrid revascularization and CABG, demonstrating at 5 years follow-up in 200 patients, similar rates of myocardial infarction, repeated revascularization, and Major Adverse Cardiac and Cerebral Events (MACCE) [13]. Repossini et al., in 2019, completed a follow-up at 15 years on more than ones thousand patients who underwent MIDCAB with a survival rate of 83% for the treatment of single-vessel disease by LIMA to LAD. Looking at these data, the isolated MIDCAB can be considered a safe and effective operation [14].

There are only two reports in the literature documenting worse outcomes of hybrid revascularization. Both of them have some flaws, either the limited number of patients or the retrospective nature coupled with relatively short follow-up. Namely, a recent one showed worse outcomes in the hybrid group at two years follow-up: Hannan et al. analyzed retrospective data from New York registries. At six years follow-up, a worse survival rate (80.9% vs. 85.8%) and repeated revascularization rate (88.2% vs. 76.6%) in the hybrid arm emerged [15]. This evaluation highlighted the very low percentage of hybrid cases, 0.8% of the total CABG procedures [16–20]. Also, in our limited series, the patients treated with the hybrid strategy represent 1.5% of the total number of CABG patients in the same period of observation. In the STS Database, the hybrid approach only represents 0.48% of the total CABG operations in North America between 2011 and 2013 [21]. Surgical advances coupled with improvements in coronary stents may broaden the application of hybrid strategies in the future.

Other recent trials that compared the results of hybrid, standard CABG, and PCI showed an incomplete revascularization rate of 7.7%, 8.0%, and 5.7% and a restenosis rate of 8.2%, 20.4%, and 5.9%, respectively. The latter despite less residual ischemia at 12 months in the hybrid group (6.4% vs. 6.7% vs. 7.9%, respectively) [21–24].

A meta-analysis comparing a hybrid coronary revascularization and PCI found a lower rate of myocardial infarction and target vessel revascularization in the hybrid group, but no difference in mortality and stroke [25]. The same results were found in a more recent study by Patel et al., where 158 matched pairs with LAD proximal complex stenosis MIDCAB and DES-PCI have equivalent nine-years survival but PCI was associated with more frequent late reinterventions [19].

In the case of two-vessel disease or multi-vessel disease, the heart team cooperation plays a fundamental role as well as the patient preference. Indeed, when the hybrid approach is considered, key aspects to be taken into account are:

- At least a left ventricular systolic function (LVEF) > 45%.
- Good lung function because of the prolonged single lung ventilation required by this minimally invasive operation.
- The risk of an intramyocardial course of the LAD and the consequent possible implication of a sternotomy conversion.
- The management of double antiplatelet therapy (DAPT), with bleeding implications after a staged surgery.

In 2014, Gasior et al. conducted a feasibility study in a cohort of two hundred patients who had undergone hybrid revascularization in a two-stage fashion; the PCI was performed after 24 h from the MIDCAB operation. They observed a sternotomy conversion of 6.1%, but no major bleeding complications (2.0%) [20]. More recently, the HYBRID-COR feasibility study based on a concomitant procedure by means of Endoscopic Coronary Artery Bypass (ECAB) and PCI on DAPT in a hybrid operating room on 30 patients showed only one chest revision for bleeding and one death at more than 4 years follow-up [22]. The management of DAPT represents a key point in the hybrid strategy for myocardial revascularization. In our hybrid series, 5 out of 14 patients underwent PCI during the same hospitalization but in a two-stage fashion, not concomitantly, without facing bleeding complications that required surgical revision. Indeed, the optimal treatment protocols are still debated: two-stage coronary revascularization ensures optimal results and does not require a hybrid operating room. However, they could face a risk of ischemia originating from non-LAD territories during the surgical grafting and a cumulative risk (negligible) of repeated reintervention if the percutaneous approach fails. On the other hand, patients undergoing PCI before surgery could have a risk of stent thrombosis, increased peri- and post-operative bleeding due to dual antiplatelet therapy (although this issue was satisfactory in our series, thanks to careful Multiplate analysis and Cangrelor Embrication), along with complications in the LAD territory during the separating time interval [23]. Last, the anastomosis is not evaluated in angiography if the PCI is performed as the first step. Although with limited evidence [24], all these issues could be overcome with a one-stage hybrid procedure protocol. The procedure requires that the hybrid room and the entire operating team must be experienced, ensuring that the PCI to high-risk non-LAD lesions can be safely performed with a protected anterior territory, and conventional CABG remains an option in cases of unsuccessful stent implantation. Moreover, surgical anastomosis can be studied before performing PCI.

The results of the STS database reported a reoperation for bleeding in 3.6% and 2.4% for a concomitant and two-stage procedure, respectively, with a mortality rate of 3.6% vs. 1.4% [21]. Repossini et al. compared the rate of reoperation for bleeding in the single MIDCAB group and a two-stage hybrid group and it resulted in 1.5% and 2.5%, respectively; a bleeding amount of more than 1000 mL that did not require reoperation was remarkable too (1.2% vs. 4.5%) [18]. The MERGING trial that compared 40 hybrids with a PCI performed 48–72 h after operation, and 20 CABG patients showed bleeding rates of 7.5% and 5.0%, respectively, although this was not statistically significant [19].

Actually, there is no evidence in those limited reports in the literature that HCR provides better results than traditional CABG or PCI in multivessel disease, and for this reason, there are nowadays no guidelines. We will be able to improve the results with the use of multiple arterial grafts and next-generation stents. A hybrid approach can be considered a viable option in myocardial revascularization when solid cooperation between cardiologists and cardiac surgeons is established, with careful attention to indications, limitations, and management, because not every patient is suitable for HCR. An ongoing multicenter randomized trial will confirm the quality of life and recovery between MIDCAB and standard sternotomy CABG the MIST Trial [25]. This study will eventually corroborate the very good outcomes of Mid-CAB in the long term (more than 20 years) when performed in a carefully selected patient population [26–28]. Robotic iterations of this operation are already performed in leading centers worldwide, aiming to establish the maximal level of a true minimally invasive approach and providing good long-term outcomes in patients who are not candidates for conventional CABG [29].

5. Study Limitations

The study has some drawbacks to disclose. First, it is a single-center feasibility report, without a control group (the HCR group separately reports its outcomes in a longitudinal way, within the isolated overall MIDCAB, not as a comparative analysis) and the analyzed sample is relatively small. Although all the HCR patients underwent a control coronary angiography, no routine coronary angiography was performed in asymptomatic patients treated with isolated MIDCAB during follow-up.

6. Conclusions

Isolated MIDCAB and hybrid revascularization are associated with encouraging short- and long-term results in appropriately selected patients. All these evaluations should be made within the heart team based on clinical presentation and on individual coronary anatomy. The staging of the indexed procedure can differ and a certain flexibility concerning the technical variables is advisable given the good surgical outcomes when a double antiplatelet therapy is adopted. Complete revascularization should be the cornerstone independent of the strategy adopted.

Author Contributions: Conceptualization, T.T., A.P., M.V. and S.D.; methodology, T.T. and A.P.; software, T.T. and F.T.; validation, E.F., G.P. and S.D. investigation, T.T., A.P. and L.A.L.; writing—original draft preparation, T.T. and A.P.; writing—review and editing, M.V., M.M. and S.B.; visualization, F.T. and L.A.L.; supervision, M.V., E.F., G.P. and S.D. All authors have read and agreed to the published version of the manuscript.

Funding: This research received no external funding.

Institutional Review Board Statement: The study was conducted according to the privacy policy of the Cardiocentro Ticino Institute and the internal regulations for the appropriate use of anonymized data in patient-oriented research, which are based on international regulations, including the Declaration of Helsinki (MEC-2020-0454). All patients signed informed consent forms for surgery and the Ethics Committee of Canton of Ticino approved the study design (CE 3103/BASEC 2016-0519, approval date: 22 March 2017).

Informed Consent Statement: Informed consent was obtained from all subjects involved in the study.

Data Availability Statement: Available by request to the Authors.

Acknowledgments: The authors wish to express their gratitude to Chantal Zurfluh for her invaluable contribution.

Conflicts of Interest: The authors declare no conflicts of interest.

References

1. Favaloro, R.G.; Effler, D.B.; Groves, L.K.; Sones FMJr Fergusson, D.J. Myocardial revascularization by internal mammary artery implant procedures. *Clin. Exp. J. Thorac. Cardiovasc. Surg.* **1967**, *54*, 359–370. [CrossRef] [PubMed]
2. Ruel, M.; Shariff, M.A.; Lapierre, H.; Goyal, N.; Dennie, C.; Sadel, S.M.; Sohmer, B.; McGinn, J.T., Jr. Results of the Minimally Invasive Coronary Artery Bypass Grafting Angiographic Patency Study. *J. Thorac. Cardiovasc. Surg.* **2014**, *147*, 203–208. [CrossRef] [PubMed]
3. Bonaros, N.; Schachner, T.; Kofler, M.; Lehr, E.; Lee, J.; Vesely, M.; Zimrin, D.; Feuchtner, G.; Friedrich, G.; Bonatti, J. Advanced hybrid closed chest revascularization: An innovative strategy for the treatment of multivessel coronary artery disease. *Eur. J. Cardiothorac. Surg.* **2014**, *46*, e94–e102; discussion e102. [CrossRef] [PubMed]
4. McGinn Jr, J.T.; Usman, S.; Lapierre, H.; Pothula, V.R.; Mesana, T.G.; Ruel, M. Minimally invasive coronary artery bypass grafting: Dual-center experience in 450 consecutive patients. *Circulation* **2009**, *120* (Suppl. S11), S78–S84. [CrossRef] [PubMed]
5. Head, S.J.; Davierwala, P.M.; Serruys, P.W.; Redwood, S.R.; Colombo, A.; Mack, M.J.; Morice, M.C.; Holmes, D.R., Jr.; Feldman, T.E.; Ståhle, E. Coronary artery bypass grafting vs. percutaneous coronary intervention for patients with three-vessel disease: Final five-year follow-up of the SYNTAX trial. *Eur. Heart J.* **2014**, *35*, 2821–2830. [CrossRef]
6. D'Ascenzo, F.; Iannaccone, M.; Saint-Hilary, G.; Bertaina, M.; Schulz-Schüpke, S.; Wahn Lee, C.; Chieffo, A.; Helft, G.; Gili, S.; Barbero, U.; et al. Impact of design of coronary stents and length of dual antiplatelet therapies on ischemic and bleeding events: A network meta-analysis of 64 randomized controlled trials and 102735 patients. *Eur. Heart J.* **2017**, *38*, 3160–3172. [CrossRef]
7. Neumann, F.J.; Sousa-Uva, M.; Ahlsson, A.; Alfonso, F.; Banning, A.P.; Benedetto, U.; Byrne, R.A.; Collet, J.P.; Falk, V.; Head, S.J.; et al. 2018 ESC/EACTS Guidelines on myocardial revascularization. *Eur. Heart J.* **2019**, *40*, 87–165. [CrossRef] [PubMed]
8. Blaas, I.; Heinz, K.; Würtinger, P.; Türkcan, A.; Tepeköylü, C.; Grimm, M.; Doppler, C.; Danzl, K.; Messner, B.; Bernhard, D. Vein graft thrombi, a niche for smooth muscle cell colonization—A hypothesis to explain the asymmetry of intimal hyperplasia. *J. Thromb. Haemost.* **2016**, *14*, 1095–1104. [CrossRef]
9. Writing Committee Members; Hillis, L.D.; Smith, P.K.; Anderson, J.L.; Bittl, J.A.; Bridges, C.R.; Byrne, J.G.; Cigarroa, J.E.; DiSesa, V.J.; Hiratzka, L.F.; et al. 2011 ACCF/AHA Guideline for Coronary Artery Bypass Graft Surgery. A report of the American College of Cardiology Foundation/American Heart Association Task Force on Practice Guidelines. *Circulation* **2011**, *124*, e652–e735. [CrossRef] [PubMed]
10. Writing Committee Members; Lawton, J.S.; Tamis-Holland, J.E.; Bangalore, S.; Bates, E.R.; Beckie, T.M.; Bischoff, J.M.; Bittl, J.A.; Cohen, M.G.; DiMaio, J.M.; et al. 2021 ACC/AHA/SCAI Guideline for Coronary Artery Revascularization. A report of the American College of Cardiology/American Heart Association Joint Committee on Practice Guidelines. *Circulation* **2022**, *145*, e18–e114. [CrossRef]
11. Moreno, P.R.; Stone, G.W.; Gonzales-Lengua, C.A.; Puskas, J.D. The hybrid coronary approach for optimal revascularization. *J. Am. Coll. Cardiol.* **2020**, *76*, 321–333. [CrossRef]
12. Raja, S.G.; Uzzaman, M.; Garg, S.; Santhirakumaran, G.; Lee, M.; Soni, M.K.; Khan, H. Comparison of minimally invasive direct coronary artery bypass and drug-eluting stents for management of isolated left anterior descending artery disease: A systematic review and meta-analysis of 7710 patients. *Ann. Cardiothorac. Surg.* **2018**, *7*, 567–576. [CrossRef]
13. Tajstra, M.; Hrapkowicz, T.; Hawranek, M.; Filipiak, K.; Gierlotka, M.; Zembala, M.; Gąsior, M.; Zembala, M.O.; POL-MIDES Study Investigators. Hybrid coronary revascularization in selected patients with multivessel disease: 5-year clinical outcomes of the prospective randomized pilot study. *JACC Cardiovasc. Interv.* **2018**, *11*, 847–852. [CrossRef]
14. Repossini, A.; Di Bacco, L.; Nicoli, F.; Passaretti, B.; Stara, A.; Jonida, B.; Muneretto, C. Minimally invasive coronary artery bypass: Twenty-year experience. *J. Thorac. Cardiovasc. Surg.* **2019**, *158*, 127–138. [CrossRef]
15. Hannan, E.L.; Wu, Y.; Cozzens, K.; Sundt, T.M., 3rd; Girardi, L.; Chikwe, J.; Wechsler, A.; Smith, C.R.; Gold, J.P.; Lahey, S.J.; et al. Hybrid coronary revascularization versus conventional coronary artery bypass surgery: Utilization and comparative outcomes. *Circ. Cardiovasc. Interv.* **2020**, *13*, e009386. [CrossRef]
16. Esteves, V.; Oliveira, M.A.; Feitosa, F.S.; Mariani, J., Jr.; Campos, C.M.; Hajjar, L.A.; Lisboa, L.A.; Jatene, F.B.; Filho, R.K.; Lemos Neto, P.A. Late clinical outcomes of myocardial hybrid revascularization versus coronary artery bypass grafting for complex triple-vessel disease: Long-term follow-up of the randomized MERGING clinical trial. *Catheter. Cardiovasc. Interv.* **2021**, *97*, 259–264. [CrossRef]
17. Ganyukov, V.; Kochergin, N.; Shilov, A.; Tarasov, R.; Skupien, J.; Szot, W.; Kokov, A.; Popov, V.; Kozyrin, K.; Barbarash, O.; et al. Randomized clinical trial of surgical vs. percutaneous vs. hybrid revascularization in multivessel coronary artery disease: Residual myocardial ischemia and clinical outcomes at one year-Hybrid. coronary REvascularization versus Stenting or Surgery (HREVS). *J. Interv. Cardiol.* **2020**, *3*, 5458064. [CrossRef]
18. Van den Eynde, J.; Sá, M.P.; De Groote, S.; Amabile, A.; Sicouri, S.; Ramlawi, B.; Torregrossa, G.; Oosterlinck, W. Hybrid coronary revascularization versus percutaneous coronary intervention: A systematic review and meta-analysis. *IJC Heart Vasc.* **2021**, *37*, 100916. [CrossRef]
19. Patel, N.C.; Hemli, J.M.; Seetharam, K.; Singh, V.P.; Scheinerman, S.J.; Pirelli, L.; Brinster, D.R.; Kim, M.C. Minimally invasive coronary bypass versus percutaneous coronary intervention for isolated complex stenosis of the left anterior descending coronary artery. *J. Thorac. Cardiovasc. Surg.* **2022**, *163*, 1839–1846. [CrossRef]

20. Gąsior, M.; Zembala, M.O.; Tajstra, M.; Filipiak, K.; Gierlotka, M.; Hrapkowicz, T.; Hawranek, M.; Poloński, L.; Zembala, M.; POL-MIDES (HYBRID) Study Investigators. Hybrid revascularization for multivessel coronary artery disease. *JACC Cardiovasc. Interv.* **2014**, *7*, 1277–1283. [CrossRef]
21. Harskamp, R.E.; Brennan, J.M.; Xian, Y.; Halkos, M.E.; Puskas, J.D.; Thourani, V.H.; Gammie, J.S.; Taylor, B.S.; de Winter, R.J.; Kim, S.; et al. Practice patterns and clinical outcomes after hybrid coronary revascularization in the United States: An analysis from the society of thoracic surgeons adult cardiac database. *Circulation* **2014**, *130*, 872–879. [CrossRef]
22. Sanetra, K.; Buszman, P.P.; Jankowska-Sanetra, J.; Cisowski, M.; Fil, W.; Gorycki, B.; Bochenek, A.; Slabon-Turska, M.; Konopko, M.; Kaźmierczak, P.; et al. One-stage hybrid coronary revascularization for the treatment of multivessel coronary artery disease-Periprocedural and long-term results from the "HYBRID-COR" feasibility study. *Front. Cardiovasc. Med.* **2022**, *9*, 1016255. [CrossRef]
23. Panoulas, V.F.; Colombo, A.; Margonato, A.; Maisano, F. Hybrid coronary revascularization: Promising, but yet to take off. *J. Am. Coll. Cardiol.* **2015**, *65*, 85–97. [CrossRef]
24. Manuel, L.; Fong, L.S.; Betts, K.; Bassin, L.; Wolfenden, H. LIMA to LAD grafting returns patient survival to age-matched population: 20-year outcomes of MIDCAB surgery. *Interact. Cardiovasc. Thorac. Surg.* **2022**, *35*, ivac243. [CrossRef]
25. Guo, M.H.; Wells, G.A.; Glineur, D.; Fortier, J.; Davierwala, P.M.; Kikuchi, K.; Lemma, M.G.; Mishra, Y.K.; McGinn, J.; Ramchandani, M.; et al. Minimally Invasive coronary surgery compared to STernotomy coronary artery bypass grafting: The MIST trial. *Contemp. Clin. Trials* **2019**, *78*, 140–145. [CrossRef] [PubMed]
26. Shimamura, J.; Miyamoto, Y.; Hibino, M.; Fukuhara, S.; Takayama, H.; Itagaki, S.; Takagi, H.; Kuno, T. Long-Term Outcomes After Hybrid Coronary Revascularization Versus Coronary Artery Bypass Grafting: Meta-Analysis of Kaplan-Meier-Derived Data. *Am. J. Cardiol.* **2024**, *212*, 13–22. [CrossRef]
27. Nagraj, S.; Tzoumas, A.; Kakargias, F.; Giannopoulos, S.; Ntoumaziou, A.; Kokkinidis, D.G.; Alvarez Villela, M.; Latib, A. Hybrid coronary revascularization (HCR) versus coronary artery bypass grafting (CABG) in multivessel coronary artery disease (MVCAD): A meta-analysis of 14 studies comprising 4226 patients. *Catheter Cardiovasc. Interv.* **2022**, *100*, 1182–1194. [CrossRef]
28. Demirsoy, E.; Mavioglu, I.; Dogan, E.; Gulmez, H.; Dindar, I.; Erol, M.K. The Feasibility and Early Results of Multivessel Minimally Invasive Coronary Artery Bypass Grafting for All Comers. *J. Clin. Med.* **2023**, *12*, 5663. [CrossRef]
29. Dokollari, A.; Sicouri, S.; Erten, O.; Gray, W.A.; Shapiro, T.A.; McGeehin, F.; Badri, M.; Coady, P.; Gnall, E.; Caroline, M.; et al. Long-term clinical outcomes of robotic-assisted surgical coronary artery revascularisation. *EuroIntervention* **2024**, *20*, 45–55. [CrossRef]

Disclaimer/Publisher's Note: The statements, opinions and data contained in all publications are solely those of the individual author(s) and contributor(s) and not of MDPI and/or the editor(s). MDPI and/or the editor(s) disclaim responsibility for any injury to people or property resulting from any ideas, methods, instructions or products referred to in the content.

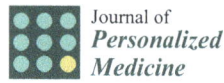

Brief Report

The Role of Myocardial Perfusion Imaging in the Prediction of Major Adverse Cardiovascular Events at 1 Year Follow-Up: A Single Center's Experience

Paraskevi Zotou [1], Aris Bechlioulis [2], Spyridon Tsiouris [1], Katerina K. Naka [2,*], Xanthi Xourgia [1], Konstantinos Pappas [2], Lampros Lakkas [2], Aidonis Rammos [2], John Kalef-Ezra [1], Lampros K. Michalis [2] and Andreas Fotopoulos [1]

[1] Nuclear Medicine Department, University Hospital of Ioannina, 45500 Ioannina, Greece
[2] Second Department of Cardiology, Faculty of Medicine, School of Health Sciences, University of Ioannina and University Hospital of Ioannina, 45500 Ioannina, Greece; md02798@yahoo.gr (A.B.)
* Correspondence: drkknaka@gmail.com; Tel.: +30-26-5100-7710

Abstract: Background: Myocardial perfusion imaging via single-photon emission computed tomography (SPECT MPI) is a well-established method of diagnosing coronary artery disease (CAD). The purpose of this study was to assess the role of SPECT MPI in predicting major cardiovascular events. Methods: The study population was composed of 614 consecutive patients (mean age: 67 years, 55% male) referred for SPECT MPI due to symptoms of stable CAD. The SPECT MPI was performed using a single-day protocol. We conducted a follow-up on all patients at 12 months via a telephone interview. Results: The majority of our patients (78%) presented findings suggestive of reversible ischemia, fixed defects or both. Extensive perfusion defects were found in 18% of the population, while LV dilation was found in 7%. During the 12-month follow-up, 16 deaths, 8 non-fatal MIs and 20 non-fatal strokes were recorded. There was no significant association of SPECT findings with the combined endpoint of all-cause death, non-fatal MI and non-fatal stroke. The presence of extensive perfusion defects was an independent predictor of mortality at 12 months (HR: 2.90, 95% CI: 1.05, 8.06, $p = 0.041$). Conclusions: In a high-risk patient population with suspected stable CAD, only large reversible perfusion defects in SPECT MPI were independently associated with mortality at 1 year. Further trials are needed to validate our findings and refine the role of SPECT MPI findings in the diagnosis and prognosis of cardiovascular patients.

Keywords: myocardial perfusion imaging; SPECT study; coronary artery disease; mortality; major adverse cardiovascular events

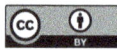

1. Introduction

Cardiovascular disease (CVD) is the leading cause of death in the western world, and coronary artery disease (CAD) is the most common form of CVD [1]. Patients with symptoms suggestive of CAD undergo a series of evaluations based on their relevant risk, ultimately assessing the need for invasive coronary angiography and the need for treatment. Diagnostic methods for coronary artery disease provide information both on the presence of angiographically significant CAD and also on the clinical prognosis of patients (i.e., mortality, non-fatal myocardial infarction, angina, etc.) [2].

Myocardial perfusion imaging (MPI) via single-photon emission computed tomography (SPECT) is a well-established nuclear cardiology method used to assess the coronary artery blood supply of the left ventricle. Performed in conjunction with a stress test (physical or pharmacological), SPECT MPI is a valuable imaging modality used to diagnose CAD, allowing for the evaluation of the extent and severity of CAD as assessed via coronary angiography [3]. The diagnostic performance of SPECT MPI has been extensively studied, with considerable heterogeneity in the estimated accuracy among studies [4]. Whether

SPECT MPI findings may further improve patient risk stratification and determine the occurrence of major clinical events is still a matter of debate [3,5].

The aim of the current single-center study was to evaluate the prognostic role of SPECT MPI, in terms of predicting mortality and other major cardiovascular events at 1 year, in symptomatic patients assessed for suspected stable CAD in the modern era.

2. Patients and Methods

2.1. Study Population

The study population consisted of 614 patients referred for SPECT MPI in the Nuclear Medicine Department of a tertiary hospital over a year (1 January to 31 December 2017) due to symptoms (i.e., chest pain (CCS class I or II) or dyspnea (NYHA class I-III)) suggestive of suspected stable CAD. Patients who needed a revascularization procedure according to the MPI study results were retrospectively excluded from our analysis. A revascularization procedure based on the reference SPECT MPI study results may have an important impact on the prognosis of the patients and would complicate the association of SPECT MPI findings with the clinical outcomes. Other exclusion criteria were: a recent myocardial infarction (MI) in the last month before the test or a coronary revascularization procedure (percutaneous coronary intervention or coronary artery bypass graft) in the last two months.

2.2. Study Protocol

On the day of the test, every patient was interviewed to enable us to record all the data relevant to their cardiovascular history. This information involved cardiac-related symptoms, risk factors for CAD (smoking habits, hypertension, diabetes mellitus, dyslipidemia, obesity, family history of CAD) and a previous history of any diagnosed CVD and its management. The study protocol and the SPECT MPI procedure were explained in detail to the patients, who gave their written informed consent to participate. The study was compliant with the principles of the Helsinki Declaration and with local legislation, and was approved by the Scientific Council and Ethical Committee of the hospital.

We conducted a follow-up on all patients enrolled in the study at 12 months after the SPECT MPI via a telephone interview. The patients—or their next of kin—were asked in detail about the occurrence of clinical events of importance in the time interval since their enrollment in the study. In case a major cardiovascular event was reported, the findings were confirmed via review of the corresponding medical records. The primary endpoint of the study was the composite of all-cause mortality, nonfatal MI and nonfatal stroke. MI and stroke were defined according to the clinical criteria of hospitalization, biochemical blood tests, electrocardiography and brain imaging.

2.3. Myocardial Perfusion Imaging Protocol

The same data acquisition parameters were used in all patients. SPECT MPI was performed according to the guidelines of the European Association of Nuclear Medicine and Molecular Imaging (EANMMI) [6]. The single-day protocol was used, with stress and rest images acquired in that particular order, approximately two hours apart. Patients fasted for at least four hours before the exam and abstained from methyl-xanthine beverages and caffeine for 24 h, in order to be prepared to undergo vasodilative stress with dipyridamole, if needed. Discontinuation of medications containing nitrates, calcium channel antagonists and beta-blockers was also applied for 24 h before the test.

Maximal or symptom-limited treadmill exercise (Bruce protocol) was selected for those patients who were capable of completing this type of stress test. Intravenous pharmacological stress was applied to patients with limited physical tolerance or with contraindications for treadmill exercise. In those patients, the vasodilative substance dipyridamole (0.56 mg/kg body weight) was mostly used, either alone or in combination with a single-stage 3 min Bruce treadmill exercise. In a small proportion of patients who were ineligible to receive dipyridamole, an inotropic pharmacological stress was carried out with the IV infusion of dobutamine. All studies were performed with Technetium Tc 99m tetrofosmin

(TF) (Myoview, GE Healthcare AS, Oslo, Norway), an MPI radiopharmaceutical that was labeled in-house according to the manufacturer's instructions.

2.4. Visual Analysis of Myocardial Perfusion

The recorded raw tomographic data under stress and rest were processed and reconstructed in the three planes (short axis, horizontal long axis and vertical long axis) according to established algorithms, and assessed by two experienced board-certified nuclear medicine physicians. The readers were not blinded to the clinical information and reported jointly to reach an agreement according to routine clinical reporting protocols; possible discrepancies were resolved via consensus. A perfusion study was interpreted visually as normal when bearing no or only borderline equivocal findings. The presence of reversible perfusion deficits was characterized as ischemia, while fixed (irreversible) deficits corresponded either to myocardial necrosis (scar) or to a gravely ischemic (hibernating) myocardium. Finally, studies with coexisting ischemia and irreversible deficits were characterized as having mixed deficits. Further evaluation of each SPECT study involved the estimation of the extent of abnormal left ventricular perfusion by the number of involved myocardial segments, graded on a 3-point scale as: absent or negligible (<1 segment or <5% of the left ventricular myocardium), small to medium (1–4 segments or 5–20% left ventricular myocardium) or large ($\geq$5 segments or >20% left ventricular myocardium) [7].

2.5. Statistical Analysis

Continuous data are presented as mean values $\pm$ standard deviation, while dichotomous data are presented as numbers (percentage). The association of SPECT MPI findings, as well other clinical parameters, with clinical outcomes was assessed using Cox's Regression analysis, and Hazard Ratio (HR) estimates (95% confidence interval) were calculated. In multivariate analysis, only the predictive role of SPECT features with a significant univariate association with clinical outcomes was assessed. Receiver–Operator Curve analysis was used to assess the prognostic value of perfusion defects for mortality. A two-tailed p value < 0.05 was used to determine significant associations. All analyses were performed using the software IBM SPSS Statistics version 21 (IBM, Armonk, NY, USA).

3. Results

The mean age of the population was 67 years, and most patients were male (55%). The prevalence of established cardiovascular risk factors is shown in Table 1. A history of CAD was present in 34% of our patients. Patients were referred for a SPECT MPI test due to chest pain (62%) and/or dyspnea (76%). The majority of our patients (78%) presented findings in the SPECT study that were suggestive of reversible ischemia, fixed defects or both. Extensive perfusion defects were found in 18% of the patients, while left ventricular dilation was found in only 7% of the population. Based on the SPECT results and the clinical findings, 307 (50%) patients were referred for invasive coronary angiography. The finding of extensive perfusion defects was associated with the presence of significant CAD in coronary angiography (r = 0.136, p = 0.017).

During the 12-month follow-up, 16 deaths (2.6%), 8 non-fatal MIs (1.3%) and 20 non-fatal strokes (3.3%) occurred. Of the patients who died, 50% had undergone a coronary angiogram; none of them had significant coronary artery disease. There was no significant association of SPECT findings with the primary endpoint (combined endpoint of all-cause death, non-fatal MI and non-fatal stroke) (Table 2).

Table 1. Descriptive characteristics of enrolled patients and results of myocardial perfusion imaging SPECT study.

Age, years	67 ± 10
Male gender, n (%)	340 (55)
Body mass index, kg/m^2	29.1 ± 4.8
Waist circumference, cm	111 ± 12
Chest Pain (CCS class I-II), n (%) Typical pain Atypical pain Non-angina pain	383 (62) 108 (17) 215 (35) 60 (10)
Dyspnea, n (%) Low workload—NYHA III Moderate workload—NYHA II High workload—NYHA I-II	466 (76) 340 (55) 73 (12) 53 (9)
Currently smoking, n (%)	113 (18)
Hypertension, n (%)	477 (78)
Dyslipidemia, n (%)	469 (76)
Diabetes mellitus, n (%)	205 (33)
History of coronary artery disease, n (%) History of myocardial infarction History of Percutaneous coronary interventions History of Coronary artery bypass surgery	208 (34) 115 (19) 138 (23) 46 (8)
History of atrial fibrillation, n (%)	79 (13)
History of heart failure, n (%)	38 (6)
History of stroke, n (%)	53 (9)
History of peripheral arterial disease, n (%)	75 (12)
Medications, n (%) Beta blockers ACE-I/ATIIR blockers MRA Statins Nitrates Calcium channel blockers Diuretics Antiplatelets Anticoagulants	 335 (55) 395 (64) 33 (5) 418 (68) 55 (9) 210 (34) 220 (36) 299 (49) 72 (12)
Abnormal findings in SPECT MPI study, n (%) Reversible perfusion defects only Fixed perfusion defects only Mixed findings	478 (78) 265 (43) 52 (9) 161 (26)
Extent of perfusion defects in SPECT MPI study, n (%) Small/moderate Large	 366 (60) 112 (18)
Left ventricular dilation, n (%)	42 (7)

Table 2. Univariate associations of SPECT MPI findings with clinical outcomes at 12-month follow-up.

	HR	95% CI	p Value
Combined endpoint			
Normal study	Ref.		
Reversible perfusion defects only	1.25	0.52, 3.01	0.624
Fixed perfusion defects only	1.97	0.62, 6.19	0.249
Mixed findings	1.72	0.69, 4.26	0.242
Normal study/small or moderate defects	Ref.		
Large defects	1.56	0.79, 3.03	0.204
Normal study	Ref.		
Left ventricular dilation	1.41	0.51, 3.96	0.509
Mortality			
Normal study	Ref.		
Reversible perfusion defects only	0.68	0.15, 3.04	0.614
Fixed perfusion defects only	-	-	-
Mixed findings	2.57	0.70, 9.49	0.157
Normal study/small or moderate defects	Ref.		
Large defects	3.56	1.32, 9.55	0.012
Normal study	Ref.		
Left ventricular dilation	4.74	1.53, 14.71	0.007

The presence of extensive perfusion defects and transient left ventricular dilation was significantly associated with mortality at the 12-month follow-up (Table 2 and Figure 1). After adjustment for confounders, only the presence of extensive perfusion defects remained an independent predictor of mortality at 12 months (Table 3). In the ROC analysis, the presence of large perfusion defects was associated with 1-year mortality with an AUC of 0.632, $p = 0.072$.

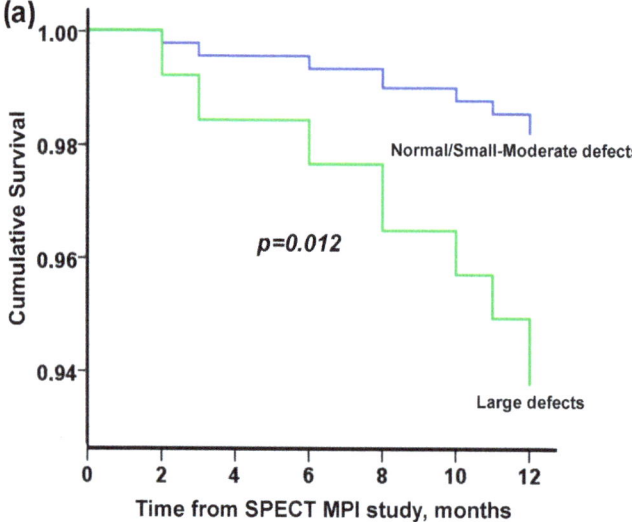

Figure 1. Cont.

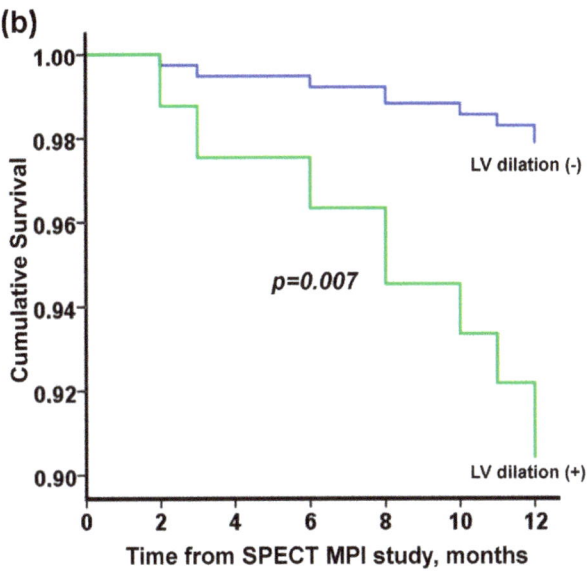

Figure 1. Cumulative survival (Kaplan–Meier curves) according to SPECT MPI study findings: (**a**) extent of defects and (**b**) presence of LV dilation.

Table 3. Associations of various studied parameters with all-cause mortality at 12-month follow-up.

	Univariate Analysis			Multivariate Analysis		
Mortality	HR	95% CI	p Value	HR	95% CI	p Value
Large defects	3.56	1.32, 9.55	0.012	2.90	1.05, 8.06	0.041
LV dilation	4.74	1.53, 14.71	0.007			
Age	1.13	1.05, 1.21	0.001	1.13	1.05, 1.22	0.001
Male gender	5.72	1.30, 25.15	0.021			
BMI	0.79	0.69, 0.90	0.001	0.80	0.68, 0.93	0.004
Waist	0.97	0.93, 1.01	0.130			
Chest pain	0.60	0.23, 1.60	0.310			
Dyspnea	1.30	0.76, 2.22	0.341			
Smoking	1.02	0.29, 3.57	0.978			
Hypertension	0.86	0.28, 2.68	0.799			
Diabetes	1.20	0.44, 3.30	0.725			
Dyslipidemia	1.34	0.38, 4.69	0.651			
History of CAD	3.28	1.19, 9.01	0.022			
Heart failure	3.60	1.03, 12.62	0.046			
History of stroke	1.49	0.34, 6.57	0.596			
Non-fatal MI						
Large defects	2.71	0.65, 11.35	0.173			
LV dilation	-	-	-			
Age	1.06	0.98, 1.16	0.150			
Male gender	1.35	0.32, 5.63	0.684			
BMI	1.08	0.95, 1.22	0.258			
Waist	1.06	1.01, 1.12	0.029	1.06	1.01, 1.12	0.029
Chest pain	0.36	0.09, 1.51	0.163			
Dyspnea	0.95	0.19, 4.70	0.948			
Smoking	0.63	0.08, 5.12	0.666			
Hypertension	0.86	0.17, 4.26	0.852			
Diabetes	1.20	0.29, 5.01	0.805			

Table 3. Cont.

	Univariate Analysis			Multivariate Analysis		
Mortality	HR	95% CI	p Value	HR	95% CI	p Value
Dyslipidemia	2.17	0.27, 17.60	0.470			
History of CAD	1.97	0.49, 7.88	0.338			
Heart failure	2.16	0.27, 17.57	0.471			
History of stroke	1.50	0.19, 12.22	0.703			
Stroke						
Large defects	0.49	0.11, 2.12	0.341			
LV dilation	-	-	-			
Age	1.08	1.02, 1.14	0.010	1.08	1.02, 1.14	0.010
Male gender	0.99	0.41, 2.38	0.975			
BMI	0.98	0.89, 1.08	0.674			
Waist	0.97	0.94, 1.01	0.134			
Chest pain	0.60	0.25, 1.43	0.247			
Dyspnea	2.87	0.67, 12.38	0.157			
Smoking	1.50	0.54, 4.12	0.435			
Hypertension	1.64	0.48, 5.59	0.430			
Diabetes	0.50	0.17, 1.48	0.208			
Dyslipidemia	1.25	0.42, 3.72	0.695			
History of CAD	1.61	0.67, 3.88	0.291			
Heart failure	1.72	0.40, 7.41	0.467			
History of stroke	2.74	0.91, 8.18	0.072			

4. Discussion

Our study involved a very high-risk cohort of consecutive symptomatic patients evaluated for suspected CAD, with almost one third of them having a history of CAD. The study patients were extensively treated with statins, antithrombotic medications and other established modern therapies for CVD. In this group of patients, we recorded a relatively high incidence of major adverse cardiovascular events and deaths (4.6% and 2.6%, respectively, at 1 year; this appears to be higher compared to some studies [8,9], although similar results have recently been reported in other studies in similar populations [10]. In the current study, the SPECT MPI findings were not found to be associated with the combined endpoint of death/non-fatal MI or stroke during a 12-month follow-up. However, a significant association of specific SPECT MPI findings (i.e., large ischemic defects and left ventricular dilatation) with all-cause mortality at 12 months was shown. After adjusting for confounders, only large ischemic defects were found to have an independent association with all-cause mortality; patients with large reversible deficits in the SPECT MPI had a ca. three times higher risk of death at 1 year compared to patients with smaller reversible deficits or no deficits.

Myocardial scintigraphy is an important tool for diagnosing CAD, and its combination with other clinical features has been suggested to lead to the more accurate stratification of prognoses and the determination of subsequent treatment policies [11]. Various recent studies have reported a significant, and probably independent, prognostic role of an abnormal SPECT MPI test in different populations, i.e., patients with diabetes mellitus, chronic kidney disease or suspected CAD, irrespective of the presence of obstructive CAD following angiography [12–16]. In these populations, the presence of a normal SPECT MPI study was associated with a lower occurrence of cardiovascular events. In the current study, only the presence of extensive ischemia was found to be related to all-cause mortality, but not to the occurrence of the combined endpoint (death, MI and stroke). The discordant associations observed among various studies may be attributed to differences in design and population characteristics, in the definitions of the endpoints of interest, as well as in the follow-up duration among studies.

Furthermore, it should be noted that different findings of the SPECT MPI study may provide important information for different outcomes. Besides the established role of fixed and reversible perfusion deficits in the diagnosis of suspected CAD, other findings, such as transient left ventricular dilatation and the presence of large reversible perfusion defects, may offer important prognostic information in terms of clinical events, and most importantly, mortality. Indeed, it has previously been shown that specific thresholds of the extent of SPECT MPI-detected ischemia may have a significant independent prognostic role, and thus, may lead to an improvement in the risk stratification of patients with suspected CAD and potential refinement of treatment in these patients [10,17–19]. The presence of transient left ventricular dilation has been associated with the diagnosis of extensive, severe CAD and poor prognosis [20]. In the absence of significant CAD, it may be a sign of severe dysfunction of the coronary microcirculation [21,22].

5. Limitations

The study was performed in a tertiary care hospital and reflects the practice settings of a single center in a specific cohort of patients, so generalizability may be limited. The exact cause of mortality was not always easy to define; thus, all-cause mortality was chosen as a clinical outcome instead of cardiovascular or other forms of cause-specific mortality. Although the SPECT MPI interpretation was performed by experienced readers, it only involved qualitative visual assessment of the left ventricular perfusion that was applied routinely in the day-to-day clinical reporting practice of this medical center.

6. Conclusions

In conclusion, in this contemporary cohort of a high-risk patient population (treated with modern treatment modalities as suggested by the guidelines) with symptoms suggestive of CAD, SPECT MPI findings of large reversible defects were independently associated with increased mortality 1 year after the study. Several aspects of the SPECT MPI study should be taken into account, not only for CAD diagnosis, but also for its prognosis in various populations. Further trials are needed to validate our findings and refine the role of SPECT MPI findings in the diagnosis and prognosis of cardiovascular patients.

Author Contributions: Conceptualization, P.Z., K.K.N., L.K.M. and A.F.; data curation, P.Z., A.B., S.T., X.X., K.P., L.L., A.R. and J.K.-E.; formal analysis, P.Z., A.B., K.K.N., S.T. and A.R.; investigation, P.Z., K.K.N., J.K.-E., L.K.M. and A.F.; methodology, P.Z., S.T., X.X., K.P., L.L., J.K.-E. and A.F.; supervision, K.K.N., L.K.M. and A.F.; writing—original draft, P.Z., A.B., S.T., K.K.N., L.K.M. and A.F. All authors have read and agreed to the published version of the manuscript.

Funding: This research received no external funding.

Institutional Review Board Statement: This study was conducted in accordance with the Declaration of Helsinki, and approved by the Institutional Review Board of the University Hospital of Ioannnina (1123/20-12-2016).

Informed Consent Statement: Informed consent was obtained from all subjects involved in the study.

Data Availability Statement: Data are available from the authors upon request.

Conflicts of Interest: The authors declare no conflict of interest.

References

1. Townsend, N.; Wilson, L.; Bhatnagar, P.; Wickramasinghe, K.; Rayner, M.; Nichols, M. Cardiovascular disease in Europe: Epidemiological update 2016. *Eur. Heart J.* **2016**, *37*, 3232–3245. [CrossRef]
2. Knuuti, J.; Wijns, W.; Saraste, A.; Capodanno, D.; Barbato, E.; Funck-Brentano, C.; Prescott, E.; Storey, R.F.; Deaton, C.; Cuisset, T.; et al. 2019 ESC Guidelines for the diagnosis and management of chronic coronary syndromes. *Eur. Heart J.* **2020**, *41*, 407–477. [CrossRef] [PubMed]
3. Shah, B.N.; Khattar, R.S.; Senior, R. The hibernating myocardium: Current concepts, diagnostic dilemmas, and clinical challenges in the post-STICH era. *Eur. Heart J.* **2013**, *34*, 1323–1336. [CrossRef] [PubMed]
4. Medical Advisory Secretariat. Single photon emission computed tomography for the diagnosis of coronary artery disease: An evidence-based analysis. *Ont. Health Technol. Assess Ser.* **2010**, *10*, 1–64.

5. Abdel Fattah, A.; Kamal, A.M.; Pancholy, S.; Ghods, M.; Russell, J.; Cassel, D.; Wasserleben, V.; Heo, J.; Iskandrian, A.S. Prognostic implications of normal exercise tomographic thallium images in patients with angiographic evidence of significant coronary artery disease. *Am. J. Cardiol.* **1994**, *74*, 769–771. [CrossRef] [PubMed]
6. Verberne, H.J.; Acampa, W.; Anagnostopoulos, C.; Ballinger, J.; Bengel, F.; De Bondt, P.; Buechel, R.R.; Cuocolo, A.; van Eck-Smit, B.L.F.; Flotats, A.; et al. EANM procedural guidelines for radionuclide myocardial perfusion imaging with SPECT and SPECT/CT: 2015 revision. *Eur. J. Nucl. Med. Mol. Imaging* **2015**, *42*, 1929–1940. [CrossRef]
7. Tilkemeier, P.L.; Bourque, J.; Doukky, R.; Sanghani, R.; Weinberg, R.L. ASNC imaging guidelines for nuclear cardiology procedures: Standardized reporting of nuclear cardiology procedures. *J. Nucl. Cardiol.* **2017**, *24*, 2064–2128. [CrossRef]
8. Betancur, J.; Otaki, Y.; Motwani, M.; Fish, M.B.; Lemley, M.; Dey, D.; Gransar, H.; Tamarappoo, B.; Germano, G.; Sharir, T.; et al. Prognostic Value of Combined Clinical and Myocardial Perfusion Imaging Data Using Machine Learning. *JACC Cardiovasc. Imaging* **2018**, *11*, 1000–1009. [CrossRef]
9. Otaki, Y.; Betancur, J.; Sharir, T.; Hu, L.H.; Gransar, H.; Liang, J.X.; Azadani, P.N.; Einstein, A.J.; Fish, M.B.; Ruddy, T.D.; et al. 5-Year Prognostic Value of Quantitative Versus Visual MPI in Subtle Perfusion Defects: Results from REFINE SPECT. *JACC Cardiovasc. Imaging* **2020**, *13*, 774–785. [CrossRef]
10. Kato, T.; Momose, M.; Uemura, Y.; Naya, M.; Matsumoto, N.; Hida, S.; Yamauchi, T.; Nakajima, T.; Suzuki, E.; Inoko, M.; et al. Association of the extent of myocardial ischemia with outcomes in patients with suspected coronary artery disease in Japan. *J. Cardiol.* **2022**, *80*, 475–481. [CrossRef]
11. Sakatani, T.; Nakajima, K.; Nishimura, T. Cardiovascular event risk estimated by myocardial perfusion SPECT combined with clinical data. *J. Cardiol.* **2021**, *80*, 64–71. [CrossRef] [PubMed]
12. Liu, L.; Abdu, F.A.; Yin, G.; Xu, B.; Mohammed, A.-Q.; Xu, S.; Lv, X.; Luo, Y.; Zu, L.; Yang, C.; et al. Prognostic value of myocardial perfusion imaging with D-SPECT camera in patients with ischemia and no obstructive coronary artery disease (INOCA). *J. Nucl. Cardiol.* **2020**, *28*, 3025–3037. [CrossRef] [PubMed]
13. Javaid, A.; Ahmed, A.I.; Han, Y.; Al Rifai, M.; Saad, J.M.; Alfawara, M.S.; Alahdab, F.; El Nihum, L.; Jimenez, Y.; Newstorm, E.; et al. Incremental prognostic value of spect over CCTA. *Int. J. Cardiol.* **2022**, *358*, 120–127. [CrossRef] [PubMed]
14. Caobelli, F.; Haaf, P.; Haenny, G.; Pfisterer, M.; Zellweger, M.J. Prognostic value of myocardial perfusion scintigraphy in asymptomatic patients with diabetes mellitus at high cardiovascular risk: 5-year follow-up of the prospective multicenter BARDOT trial. *Eur. J. Nucl. Med. Mol. Imaging* **2021**, *48*, 3512–3521. [CrossRef] [PubMed]
15. Cantoni, V.; Green, R.; Acampa, W.; Assante, R.; Zampella, E.; Nappi, C.; Gaudieri, V.; Mannarino, T.; D'Antonio, A.; Petretta, M.; et al. Prognostic value of myocardial perfusion imaging in patients with chronic kidney disease: A systematic review and meta-analysis. *J. Nucl. Cardiol.* **2022**, *29*, 141–154. [CrossRef]
16. Djaileb, L.; Seiller, A.; Canu, M.; De Leiris, N.; Martin, A.; Poujol, J.; Fraguas-Rubio, A.; Leenhardt, J.; Carabelli, A.; Calizzano, A.; et al. Prognostic value of SPECT myocardial perfusion entropy in high-risk type 2 diabetic patients. *Eur. J. Nucl. Med. Mol. Imaging* **2021**, *48*, 1813–1821. [CrossRef]
17. Hachamovitch, R.; Hayes, S.W.; Friedman, J.D.; Cohen, I.; Berman, D.S. A prognostic score for pre-diction of cardiac mortality risk after adenosine stress myocardial perfusion scintigraphy. *J. Am. Coll. Cardiol.* **2005**, *45*, 722–729. [CrossRef]
18. Chan, H.P.; Chang, C.C.; Hu, C.; Wang, W.H.; Peng, N.J.; Tyan, Y.C.; Yang, M.H. The Evaluation of Left Ventricle Ischemic Extent in Patients with Significantly Suspicious Cardiovascular Disease by (99m)Tc-Sestamibi Dynamic SPECT/CT and Myocardial Perfusion Imaging: A Head-to-Head Comparison. *Diagnostics* **2021**, *11*, 1101. [CrossRef]
19. Georgiopoulos, G.; Mavraganis, G.; Aimo, A.; Giorgetti, A.; Cavaleri, S.; Fabiani, I.; Giannoni, A.; Emdin, M.; Gimelli, A. Sex-specific associations of myocardial perfusion imaging with outcomes in patients with suspected chronic coronary syndrome. *Hellenic J. Cardiol.* **2022**. [CrossRef]
20. Alama, M.; Labos, C.; Emery, H.; Iwanochko, R.M.; Freeman, M.; Husain, M.; Lee, D.S. Diagnostic and prognostic significance of transient ischemic dilation (TID) in myocardial perfusion imaging: A systematic review and meta-analysis. *J. Nucl. Cardiol.* **2018**, *25*, 724–737. [CrossRef]
21. Emmett, L.; Ng, A.; Ha, L.; Russo, R.; Mansberg, R.; Zhao, W.; Chow, S.V.; Kritharides, L. Comparative assessment of rest and post-stress left ventricular volumes and left ventricular ejection fraction on gated myocardial perfusion imaging (MPI) and echocardiography in patients with transient ischaemic dilation on adenosine MPI: Myocardial stunning or subendocardial hypoperfusion? *J. Nucl. Cardiol.* **2012**, *19*, 735–742. [PubMed]
22. Chen, L.; Zhang, M.; Jiang, J.; Lei, B.; Sun, X. Coronary microvascular dysfunction: An important interpretation on the clinical significance of transient ischemic dilation of the left ventricle on myocardial perfusion imaging. *J. X-Ray Sci. Technol.* **2021**, *29*, 347–360. [CrossRef] [PubMed]

Disclaimer/Publisher's Note: The statements, opinions and data contained in all publications are solely those of the individual author(s) and contributor(s) and not of MDPI and/or the editor(s). MDPI and/or the editor(s) disclaim responsibility for any injury to people or property resulting from any ideas, methods, instructions or products referred to in the content.

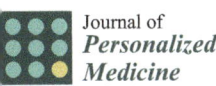

Article

Risk Factors for Acute Postoperative Delirium in Cardiac Surgery Patients >65 Years Old

Eleni Spiropoulou [1], George Samanidis [2,3,*], Meletios Kanakis [4] and Ioannis Nenekidis [2]

[1] Department of Cardiac Surgery Intensive Care, Onassis Cardiac Surgery Center, 17674 Athens, Greece
[2] Department of Adult Cardiac Surgery, Onassis Cardiac Surgery Center, 17674 Athens, Greece
[3] Onassis Cardiac Surgery Center, 356 Leoforos Syggrou, 17674 Athens, Greece
[4] Department of Pediatric and Congenital Heart Surgery, Onassis Cardiac Surgery Center, 17674 Athens, Greece
* Correspondence: gsamanidis@yahoo.gr; Tel.: +30-210-9493-833

Abstract: **Background:** Acute postoperative delirium is the most common neuropsychiatric disorder in cardiac surgery patients in the intensive care unit (ICU). The purpose of this study was to evaluate the possible risk factors of postoperative delirium (POD) for cardiac surgery patients in the ICU. **Materials and Methods:** The study population was composed of 86 cardiac surgery patients managed postoperatively in the cardiac surgery ICU. Presence of POD in patients was evaluated by the CAM-ICU scale. **Results:** According to the CAM-ICU scale, 22 (25.6%) patients presented POD; history of smoking, alcohol use, COPD, and preoperative permanent atrial fibrillation were associated with POD (for all, $p < 0.05$). The type of cardiac surgery operations, type of analgesia, and red blood cell transfusion in the ICU were not associated with POD ($p > 0.05$), while cardiac arrhythmia in the ICU, hypoxemia in the ICU after extubation ($pO_2 < 60$ mmHg), and heart rate after extubation were predisposing factors for POD (for all, $p < 0.05$). Multivariable logistic regression analysis (adjusted to risk factors) showed that hypoxemia after extubation (OR = 20.6; 95%CI: 2.82–150), heart rate after extubation (OR = 0.95; 95% CI: 0.92–0.98), and alcohol use (OR = 74.3; 95%CI: 6.41–861) were predictive factors for acute postoperative delirium (for all, $p < 0.05$). **Conclusion:** Alcohol use and respiratory dysfunction before and after heart operation were associated with acute postoperative delirium in cardiac surgery ICU patients.

Keywords: cardiac surgery; acute delirium; hypoxemia; alcohol use; intensive care unit

1. Introduction

Cognitive disorders after cardiac surgery can be presented within a spectrum of different variations in mental and emotional pathology, ranging from a mild event of temporary loss of concentration to multiple episodes of acute delirium, a condition which can jeopardize the course of a smooth postoperative outcome [1].

In fact, the term postoperative delirium (POD) is defined as temporary in most cases, and as a fluctuated disorder of consciousness presenting early in the post-surgery aftercare period. It usually appears in elderly people and in most severe heart disease patients with heavy concomitant pathology [2]. There is also a decrease in the ability to think, perceive, and recall memory, as well as intense psychomotor stimulation. The keystone symptom of POD is the disturbance of consciousness highlighted with repeated advanced alert activity just before each time the patient reaches a blurry and foggy communication environment. The classification of this neuropsychiatric condition is based on different modalities of alertness in close relation to the level of consciousness described and this basically is characterized as hyperkinetic, hypokinetic, or mixed [3].

Thus, hyperkinetic delirium is a condition of stressful behavior attached to the feeling of agony and anxiety and, in many cases, is characterized by additional elements of hallucinations and illusions. In addition, the patient may experience hallucinations (visual and auditory) and the stimulation may be due to them. The patient is usually scared and potentially aggressive. On the other side, the hypokinetic form of delirium is presented with signs of apathy, withdrawal, and leveling of emotions. The patient is usually lethargic with somnolent behavior and reduced response to stimuli. This condition resembles depression; therefore, the differential diagnosis depends on specific details derived from the psychokinetic deceleration status of the patient. Finally, the mixed type is a variety of fluctuations and transitions in between a hyper- and hypokinetic state.

The top marks of predisposing factors for developing POD include increased age, decreased cognitive function, alcohol and drug abuse, male sex, systemic adverse effects of irreversible end stage diseases, genetic predisposing, electrolyte disturbances and, potentially, depression and dementia [4–8]. The onset of POD is associated with an increased length of stay in-hospital and the ICU, postoperative rehabilitation, and mortality after discharge from the hospital, as well as the subsequent functional impoverishment of patients regardless of the presence or absence of dementia.

The purpose of this study was to evaluate the possible risk factors for POD after cardiac surgery in patients who were postoperatively treated in the ICU.

2. Patients and Methods

2.1. Study Population

The study included 86 patients who underwent cardiac surgery operations (coronary bypass grafting (CABG), heart valve surgery, or combined operations) via cardiopulmonary bypass and who were postoperatively treated in the cardiac surgery ICU. Inclusion criteria for the study were: (1) extubated patients, (2) patients with no known psychiatric disease, (3) patients could speak and understand the language, and (4) the age of patients was > 65 years old. The informed consent was obtained from the patients included in this study. This study has been approved by the Hospital Institutional Review Board (532/01-10-2014).

Present or absent POD was estimated using the confusion assessment methods-intensive care unit (CAM-ICU) scale [9]. The level of arousal and repression was measured using the Richmond Agitation-Sedation Scale (RASS), which is a 10-point scale ranging from +4 to −5, with a RASS score of 0 indicating a calm and awake patient. The diagnosis of POD was established according to the Diagnostic and Statistical Manual of Mental Disorders (DSM-IV) and if the patients met the following criteria based on the CAM-ICU scale: (1) the mental status of patients was changed acutely, accompanied with (2) inattention; (3) disorganization of thinking; or (4) an altered level of consciousness.

2.2. Statistical Analysis

Continuous variables were presented by mean ± standard deviation (SD), while nominal variables were presented by number (n) and percentage (%). The normality of the distribution of variables was evaluated using the Kolmogorov–Smirnov test and Q-Q plot. Parametric (Student's *t*-test) or non-parametric tests (Mann–Whitney test, Kruskal–Wallis test, Chi-squared test, and Fisher's exact test) were implemented for the data analysis, depending on the normality of variable distribution. Spearman (r_s) or Pearson (r) correlation tests were implemented for data analysis. Binary univariable and multivariable logistic regression analysis was implemented to identify the risk factors for POD and the effect size of risk factors to POD was expressed by odds ratio (OR). For logistic regression analysis, the Hosmer–Lemeshow test was used for goodness of fit. The confidence interval was set at 95% (95% confidence interval). The statistically significant difference was considered $p < 0.05$. IBM SPSS Statistics for Windows, version 25 (IBM Corp., Armonk, NY, USA) was used for data analysis.

3. Results

3.1. Demographic Characteristics

The study population consisted of 86 patients in which 29 patients (33.7%) were women. Regarding education, 41.9% of patients were primary school graduates while 11.6% of patients were higher education. A total of 16.3% of patients lived alone. The most common comorbidities were hypertension in 87.2% of patients and DM in 38.4% of patients. Forty-four patients had undergone previous surgery (not cardiac surgery), and 64% of patients report that they do sedentary work. Smoking and alcohol use was reported in 16.3% and 8.1% of patients, respectively. Other demographics and preoperative characteristics of patients are presented in Tables 1 and 2.

Table 1. Demographic characteristics of patients. Number = N or n.

Variable	Total Number of Patients N = 86 (%)
Gender, Woman, n (%)	29 (33.7)
Age, years old	
<74	48 (55.8)
≥75	38 (54.2)
Body mass index, n (%)	
Normal	17 (19.7)
Overweight	50 (58.1)
Obesity	19 (22.2)
Patient lives alone, n (%)	14 (16.3)
Education	
Primary	36 (41.9)
Secondary	40 (46.6)
Higher	10 (11.6)
Profession, n (%)	
Manual work	31 (36)
Sedentary work	55 (64)
Smoking	14 (16.3)
Mobility	
Good	84 (97.7)
Poor	2 (2.3)
Walking, n (%)	49 (57)
Alcohol use, n (%)	7 (8.1)
Drug use, n (%)	1 (1.2)

3.2. Perioperative Details

Regarding the type of surgery, 41.9% of patients had undergone heart valve surgery, while the most common duration of operation (3–6 h) was recorded in 51 (59.3%) patients, and the duration of CPB lasting more than 3 h was observed in 11 (12.8) patients. Regarding intraoperative blood gases, 16.3% of the patients had a pH < 7.35 and 55.9% of patients had a pH = 7.36–7.45, while in 27.8% of patients, the pH range was 7.46–7.53. As for reference pCO_2, 57% of patients had < 34 mmHg, 39.5% had 35 mmHg–45 mmHg, and 3.5% had 46 mmHg–48 mmHg. In terms of the type of analgesic administered, 64 (74.4%) patients used paracetamol + morphine, while paracetamol + morphine + midazolam were administered for 9 (10.5%) patients. According to the CAM-ICU scale, 22 (25.6%) patients postoperatively presented acute postoperative delirium in ICU. Additional perioperative details are listed in Table 2.

Table 2. Preoperative and intraoperative details. Number = N or n; chronic obstructive pulmonary disease = COPD; coronary artery bypass grafting = CABG; intensive care unit = ICU; confusion assessment methods-intensive care unit = CAM-ICU.

Variable	Total Number of Patients N = 86 (%)
Hypertension, n (%)	75 (87.2)
Diabetes mellitus, n (%)	33 (38.4)
COPD, n (%)	12 (14)
Hyperlipidemia, n (%)	31 (36)
Chronic renal insufficiency without hemodialysis, n (%)	9 (10.5)
Preoperative cardiac arrhythmia, n (%)	9 (10.5)
Thyroid disease, n(%)	16 (18.6)
Previous operation (other than cardiac surgery), n (%)	44 (51.2)
Depression	6 (7)
Type of operation, n (%) Heart valve CABG Combined	36 (41.9) 24 (27.9) 26 (30.2)
Time of operation, n (%) <3 h 3–6 h >6 h	32 (37.2) 51 (59.3) 3 (3.5)
Cardiopulmonary bypass time, n (%) <3 h >3 h	75 (87.2) 11 (12.8)
Intubation time, n (%) <24 h 24–48 h >48 h	77 (89.5) 5 (6.8) 4 (4.7)
Blood transfusion in ICU, n (%)	15 (17.4)
Cardiac arrhythmia in ICU, n (%)	23 (26.7)
Hypoxemia after extubation in ICU (pO_2 < 60 mmHg), n (%)	9 (10.5)
Acute postoperative delirium (CAM-ICU), n (%)	22 (25.6)

3.3. Comparison of Two Groups with and without Acute Postoperative Delirium

Analysis of our data showed that gender, patient age being <74 and ≥75 years old, education level, hypertension, diabetes mellitus, and patient living alone were not associated with POD (for all, $p > 0.05$) (Table 3). On the other hand, history of smoking, alcohol use, COPD, and preoperative permanent atrial fibrillation were associated with POD (for all, $p < 0.05$) (Table 3). In addition, the type of cardiac surgery operations, type of analgesia, and red blood cell transfusion were not associated with acute delirium ($p > 0.05$), while cardiac arrhythmia in the ICU, postoperative hypoxemia in the ICU after extubation (pO_2 < 60 mmHg), and heart rate were predisposing factors for acute delirium (for all, $p < 0.05$). Other intraoperative and postoperative results are shown in Table 4. A positive CAM-ICU value was associated with heart rate ($p = 0.04$), while the age of patients, intubation time in the ICU, response time, and operation time were not associated with CAM-ICU ($p > 0.05$).

Table 3. Comparison of demographic characteristics between two groups with and without acute postoperative delirium. Chronic obstructive pulmonary disease = COPD; number = N or n; standard deviation = SD. * Statistical significance $p < 0.05$.

Variables	Acute Postoperative Delirium		p-Value
	Yes N = 22 Patients (%)	No N = 64 Patients (%)	
Age, years old ± SD	74.6 ± 5.7	72.4 ± 5.3	0.11
Body mass index, kg/m^2 ± SD	27.8 ± 4.2	28.2 ± 3.5	0.69
Gender, n (%)			
Man	14 (63.6)	43 (67.2)	0.47
Woman	8 (36.4)	21 (32.8)	
Age, years old, (%)			
<74	9 (40.9)	39 (60.9)	0.08
≥75	13 (59.1)	25 (39.1)	
Body mass index, n (%)			
Normal	6 (27.3)	11 (17.2)	
Overweight	12 (54.5)	38 (59.4)	0.57
Obesity	4 (18.2)	15 (23.4)	
Patient lives alone, n (%)	3 (13.6)	11 (17.2)	0.49
Education, n (%)			
Primary-Secondary	11 (50)	29 (45.3)	0.44
Higher	11 (50)	35 (54.7)	
Profession, n (%)			
Manual work	8 (36.4)	23 (35.9)	0.58
Sedentary work	14 (63.6)	41 (64.1)	
Smoking, n (%)	7 (31.8)	7 (10.9)	0.02 *
Alcohol use, n (%)	6 (27.3)	1 (1.6)	0.001 *
Hypertension, n (%)	19 (86.4)	56 (87.5)	1.00
Diabetes mellitus, n (%)	8 (36.4)	25 (39.1)	0.82
COPD, n (%)	6 (27.3)	6 (9.4)	0.03 *
History of malignancy, n (%)	4 (18.2)	3 (4.7)	0.05
Hyperlipidemia, n (%)	9 (40.9)	22 (34.4)	0.38
Permanent atrial fibrillation, n (%)	5 (22.7)	4 (6.3)	0.02 *
Previous surgery (non-cardiac), n (%)	8 (36.4)	36 (56.3)	0.10
Carotid disease, n (%)	2 (9.1)	2 (3.1)	0.25
Chronic renal failure, n (%)	3 (13.6)	6 (9.4)	0.57

3.4. Univariable and Multivariable Logistic Regression Analysis

Univariable logistic regression analysis showed that permanent atrial fibrillation (p = 0.04, OR = 4.4; 95% CI: 1.06–18.2), smoking (p = 0.02, OR = 3.8; 95% CI: 1.15–12.5), alcohol use (p = 0.005, OR = 23.6; 95% CI: 2.65–210.4), intubation time in ICU (p = 0.02, OR = 1.04; 95% CI: 1.0–1.07), cardiac arrhythmia in the ICU (p = 0.03, OR = 3.3; 95% CI: 1.15–9.22), and hypoxemia in the ICU after extubation (pCO$_2$ < 60 mmHg) (p = 0.008, OR = 7.6; 95% CI: 1.71–33.8) were predictive factors for postoperative delirium. Multivariable regression logistic analysis evaluated the risk factors for POD. Multivariable logistic regression analysis (adjusted to risk factors) showed that hypoxemia after extubation (OR = 20.6; 95%CI: 2.82–150), heart rate after extubation (OR = 0.95; 95% CI: 0.92–0.98), and alcohol use (OR = 74.3; 95%CI: 6.41–861) were predictive factors for acute postoperative delirium (p < 0.05 for all).

Table 4. Comparison of perioperative details between two groups with and without acute postoperative delirium. Number = N or n; standard deviation = SD. * Statistical significance $p < 0.05$.

Variables	Acute Postoperative Delirium		p-Value
	Yes N = 22 Patients	No N = 64 Patients	
Type of operation, n (%) Heart valve CABG Combined	9 (40.9) 5 (22.7) 8 (36.4)	27 (42.2) 21 (32.8) 16 (25.0)	0.51
Operation time, hours ± SD	3.8 ± 1.3	3.3 ± 1	0.12
Cardiopulmonary bypass time, hours ± SD	2.0 ± 1.0	1.7 ± 0.9	0.24
pH (intraoperative) ± SD	7.4 ± 0.062	7.4 ± 0.056	0.92
pCO_2 (intraoperative), mmHg ± SD	34.5 ± 5.5	34 ± 4.4	0.70
pO_2 (intraoperative), mmHg ± SD	223.5 ± 81.1	232.1 ± 103.2	0.85
Level of K^+ (intraoperative), mmol/L ± SD	4.6 ± 0.59	4.5 ± 0.59	0.25
Level of Na^+ (intraoperative), mmol/L ± SD	135.1 ± 3.7	137 ± 4.18	0.03 *
Level of Ca^{++} (intraoperative), mmol/L ± SD	1.1 ± 0.54	1 ± 0.18	0.56
Level of Mg^{++} (intraoperative) ± SD	2.2 ± 0.62	2.3 ± 0.56	0.86
Level of glucose (intraoperative), mg/dL ± SD	147.7 ± 54.37	145.7 ± 38.04	0.61
Level of lactate (intraoperative), mmol/L ± SD	1.8 ± 0.76	2.2 ± 1.01	0.05
Intubation time in ICU, hours ± SD	23.8 ± 22.95	14.3 ± 9.21	0.18
Response time, min ± SD	3.7 ± 6.68	1.4 ± 0.73	0.07
pH (2 h after extubation) ± SD	7.4 ± 0.05	7.4 ± 0.035	0.54
pCO_2 (2 h after extubation), mmHg ± SD	39.5 ± 4.48	38.1 ± 3.44	0.24
pO_2 (2 h after extubation), mmHg ± SD	108.6 ± 28.1	113 ± 34.42	0.92
Level of K^+ (2 h after extubation), mmol/L ± SD	4.4 ± 0.37	4.4 ± 0.35	0.98
Level of Na^+ (2 h after extubation), mmol/L ±SD	140 ± 2.69	137.7 ± 13.2	0.55
Level of Ca^{++} (2 h after extubation), mmol/L ± SD	1 ± 0.2	1.1 ± 0.24	0.75
Level of Mg^{++} (2 h after extubation) ± SD	2.2 ± 0.61	2.2 ± 0.66	0.88
Level of glucose (2 h after extubation), mg/dL ± SD	176.2 ± 45.65	173.2 ± 31.24	0.87
Level of lactate (2 h after extubation), mmol/L ± SD	1.51 ± 0.74	1.7 ± 0.87	0.36
Systolic blood pressure (4 h after extubation), mmHg ± SD	132 ± 12.77	127.6 ± 12.93	0.12
Diastolic blood pressure (4 h after extubation), mmHg ± SD	61.8 ± 7.64	62.3 ± 8.75	0.93
Heart rate (4 h after extubation) ± SD	77.1 ± 26.13	86.8 ± 15.68	0.04 *
Temperature (4 h after extubation), °C ± SD	37.2 ± 0.41	42.5 ± 42.48	0.84
Hypoxemia after extubation (pO_2 < 60 mmHg), n (%) ± SD	6 (27.3)	3 (4.7)	0.008 *
Respiratory rates per minute (4 h after extubation) ± SD	19.5 ± 3.51	18.63 ± 5.02	0.40
Red blood cells transfusion in ICU, n (%)	2 (9.1)	13 (20.3)	0.23
Cardiac arrhythmia in ICU, n (%)	10 (45.5)	13 (20.3)	0.02 *

4. Discussion

The onset of acute postoperative delirium (POD) in ICU patients concerns the health professionals who are caring for these patients. Spear reported an increased risk of mortality; institutionalization; and dementia; independent of age; and comorbidities in patients who had versus who did not have delirium, and the mean duration of observation was

22.7 months [10]. In patients with existing disorders of cognitive functions, the rate of delirium developed with high risk and accounted for approximately in 22–89% of patients [11]. A range of 15–35% of patients presenting with POD belonged to the elderly group [12]. In the intensive care units, much higher rates of delirium have been observed, ranging from 70% to 87% of patients [6]. In addition, in patients with malignant diseases, the chances of developing delirium during the course of the disease are 11–35%, while in the final stages of the disease (as in the last weeks of life), in severe clinical conditions, its occurrence is the most common complication, which reaches 85–88% [13]. The same high percentage of 88% is observed in palliative care units of the general type [14]. In the present study, with a sample of 86 cardiac surgery patients, an attempt was made to investigate, analyze, and detect the predisposing factors that contribute to the occurrence of acute POD. According to our results, 25.6% of patients developed acute POD. On the other hand, many studies have reported that POD affects the long-term survival of patients who have undergone cardiac surgery. Gottesman et al. found that the survival rate (over 10 years) of cardiac surgery patients without POD was higher than the patients with delirium [15].

Different risk factors present to predict and identify POD and among these are alcohol use, chronic obstructive disease, smoking, number of drugs used, electrolyte disturbance, and type of anesthesia used [4,8,16].

Regarding alcohol use, it seems to be positively correlated with POD surgery patients. The results of one study showed higher rates of POD in the user group [8]. Chronic obstructive pulmonary disease is a respiratory disease with its main feature being the obstruction of the airways of the respiratory system resulting in shortness of breath and hypoxemia. Hypoxemia can lead to decreased acetylcholine levels, making individuals susceptible to delirium. In the present study, it appears to be a predisposing risk factor for acute postoperative delirium. Similarly, Szylińska et al. investigated predisposing risk factors for delirium in cardiac surgery patients, namely preoperative COPD. They revealed that 22.97% of patients with COPD were diagnosed with POD and they concluded that COPD is an important predisposing risk factor for the development of POD in cardiac surgery patients [17]. In our study, for the patients with preoperative COPD, postoperative delirium was diagnosed in 27.3% of patients, with 9.4% of patients not experiencing delirium ($p < 0.05$).

Postoperative hyponatremia appears to be positively associated with the occurrence of acute POD. This conclusion agrees with Smutler et al. in a prospective study of 142 patients (≥ 70 years) who underwent cardiac surgery [18]. They found that sodium concentration was associated with delirium. The same results were presented by Onuma et al. in patients who underwent spinal surgery at ages > 75 years old [19]. Regarding the type and number of anesthetics administered in the present study, it does not appear to be a predisposing factor for the occurrence of acute postoperative delirium. In addition, no difference in POD was observed in a study by Shin et al. that enrolled 534 cardiac surgery patients [20]. The study showed that sevoflurane with dexmedetomidine and propofol did not affect the development of POD. A recent randomized controlled trial by Momeni et al. presented no benefits of combining propofol plus dexmedetomidine versus propofol alone to prevent POD in cardiac surgery patients [21]. On the other hand, Subramanian et al. presented in their study that postoperative analgesia by postoperative intravenous acetaminophen administration combined with propofol or dexmedetomidine reduced in-hospital delirium [1]. Reports have been made of the effect of nicotine on chronic smokers and its association with delirium. According to the results of the study, chronic smokers are more likely to develop postoperative delirium due to nicotine dependence and abrupt cessation, which is consistent with the results of a study by Galyfos et al. [22]. Miyazaki et al. identified that smoking is a predisposing factor for POD in patients who underwent off-pump CABG [23]. In our study, smoking was associated with POD ($p = 0.03$).

The results from the postoperative evaluation of patients in terms of heart rate showed that arrhythmia was positively associated with the occurrence of acute postoperative delirium [24]. A consequence of arrhythmia, particularly the bradycardia, is a low cardiac output syndrome and cerebral hypoperfusion with hypoxemia. There were different types of bradycardias encountered postoperatively. These were usually sinus bradycardia, atrial fibrillation with low frequency, nodal rhythm, and second and third degree atrioventricular block. The causes of bradycardia can be varied, such as heart attack or ischemia, heart valve replacement, ASD correction, electrolyte disturbances, or even pharmacological etiology. Sometimes the consequence of bradycardia was hemodynamic instability with severe hypotension (SAP < 80 mmHg). In conclusion, bradycardia presenting in patients as a postoperative complication with consequent low cardiac output was a predisposing factor for the occurrence of POD [25].

5. Study Limitations

The small number of patients included in this study may affect our results and possible risk factors may have been underestimated. In addition, it is a single-center study and focuses on ICU patients. All patients included in this study were only cardiac surgery patients and extracted results should not be adapted for ICU patients with other pathologies in the general population. All patients underwent cardiac surgery via cardiopulmonary bypass and alcohol abuse was not recorded in the study population.

6. Conclusions

After analyzing our data, we concluded that preoperative COPD, smoking, and alcohol use were predisposing factors for the appearance of POD in ICU patients who underwent cardiac surgery operations.

Author Contributions: Conceptualization, E.S. and G.S.; Data curation, G.S.; Formal analysis, G.S.; Investigation, E.S., G.S.s, M.K. and I.N.; Methodology, E.S., M.K. and I.N.; Software, G.S.; Supervision, G.S.; Validation, G.S.; Visualization, G.S. and M.K.; Writing – original draft, E.S., G.S., M.K. and I.N. All authors have read and agreed to the published version of the manuscript.

Funding: This research received no external funding.

Institutional Review Board Statement: The study was conducted in accordance with the Declaration of Helsinki, and approved by the Institutional Review Board of Onassis Cardiac Surgery Center (532/01-10-2014).

Informed Consent Statement: Informed consent was obtained from all subjects involved in the study.

Data Availability Statement: Data available from the authors upon request.

Acknowledgments: The authors want to thank the Onassis Foundation and Onassis Cardiac Surgery Center (Athens, Greece).

Conflicts of Interest: The authors declare no conflict of interest. The funders had no role in the design of the study; in the collection, analyses, or interpretation of data; in the writing of the manuscript, or in the decision to publish the results.

References

1. Subramaniam, B.; Shankar, P.; Shaefi, S.; Mueller, A.; O'Gara, B.; Banner-Goodspeed, V.; Gallagher, J.; Gasangwa, D.; Patxot, M.; Pack-iasabapathy, S.; et al. Effect of Intravenous Acetaminophen vs Placebo Com-bined With Propofol or Dexmedetomidine on Postoperative Delirium among Older Patients Following Cardiac Surgery: The DEXACET Randomized Clinical Trial. *JAMA* **2019**, *321*, 686–696. [CrossRef]
2. lvarez-Fernandez, B.; Formiga, F.; Gomez, R. Delirium in hospitalized older persons. *J. Nutr.* **2008**, *12*, 246–251.
3. Bilotta, F.; Lauretta, M.P.; Borozdina, A.; Mizikov, V.M.; Rosa, G. Postoperative delirium: Risk factors, diagnosis and perioperative care. *Minerva Anestesiol.* **2013**, *79*, 1066–1076.
4. Aldemir, M.; Özen, S.; Kara, I.H.; Sir, A.; Baç, B. Predisposing factors for delirium in the surgical intensive care unit. *Crit. Care* **2001**, *5*, 265–270. [CrossRef]
5. Mantz, J.; Hemmings, H.C.; Boddaert, J. Case Scenario: Postoperative Delirium in Elderly Surgical Patients. *Anesthesiology* **2010**, *112*, 189–195. [CrossRef]
6. Barr, J.; Fraser, G.L.; Puntillo, K.; Ely, E.W.; Gélinas, C.; Dasta, J.F.; Davidson, J.E.; Devlin, J.W.; Kress, J.P.; Joffe, A.M.; et al. American Col-lege of Critical Care Medicine. Clinical practice guidelines for the management of pain, agitation, and delirium in adult pa-tients in the intensive care unit. *Crit. Care Med.* **2013**, *41*, 263–306. [CrossRef]

7. Lelis, R.G.B.; Krieger, J.E.; Pereira, A.C.; Schmidt, A.P.; Carmona, M.J.; Oliveira, S.A.; Auler, J.O.C. Apolipoprotein E4 genotype increases the risk of postoperative cognitive dysfunction in patients undergoing coronary artery bypass graft surgery. *J. Cardiovasc. Surg.* **2006**, *47*, 451–456.
8. Ouimet, S.; Kavanagh, B.P.; Gottfried, S.B.; Skrobik, Y. Incidence, risk factors and consequences of ICU delirium. *Intensiv. Care Med.* **2006**, *33*, 66–73. [CrossRef]
9. Khan, B.A.; Perkins, A.J.; Gao, S.; Hui, S.L.; Campbell, N.L.; Farber, M.O.; Chlan, L.L.; Boustani, M.A. The Confusion Assessment Method for the ICU-7 Delirium Severity Scale: A Novel Delirium Severity Instrument for Use in the ICU. *Crit. Care Med.* **2017**, *45*, 851–857. [CrossRef]
10. Spear, L. The adolescent brain and age-related behavioral manifestations. *Neurosci. Biobehav. Rev.* **2000**, *24*, 417–463. [CrossRef]
11. Casey, B.J.; Tottenham, N.; Liston, C.; Durston, S. Imaging the developing brain: What have we learned about cognitive develop-ment? *Trends Cogn. Sci.* **2005**, *9*, 104–110. [CrossRef]
12. Marquis, S.; Moore, M.M.; Howieson, D.B.; Sexton, G.; Payami, H.; Kaye, J.A.; Camicioli, R. Independent predictors of cognitive de-cline in healthy elderly persons. *Arch. Neurol.* **2002**, *59*, 601–606. [CrossRef]
13. Bressler, S.L. Large-scale cortical networks and cognition. *Brain Res. Rev.* **1995**, *20*, 288–304. [CrossRef]
14. Varela, F.; Lachaux, J.-P.; Rodriguez, E.; Martinerie, J. The brainweb: Phase synchronization and large-scale integration. *Nat. Rev. Neurosci.* **2001**, *2*, 229–239. [CrossRef]
15. Gottesman, R.F.; Grega, M.A.; Bailey, M.M.; Pham, L.D.; Zeger, S.L.; Baumgartner, W.A.; Selnes, O.A.; McKhann, G.M. Delirium after coronary artery bypass graft surgery and late mortality. *Ann. Neurol.* **2009**, *67*, 338–344. [CrossRef]
16. Bekker, A.Y.; Weeks, E.J. Cognitive function after anaesthesia in the elderly. *Best Pract. Res. Clin. Anaesthesiol.* **2003**, *17*, 259–272. [CrossRef]
17. Szylińska, A.; Rotter, I.; Listewnik, M.; Lechowicz, K.; Brykczyński, M.; Dzidek, S.; Żukowski, M.; Kotfis, K. Postoperative Delirium in Patients with Chronic Obstructive Pulmonary Disease after Coronary Artery Bypass Grafting. *Medicina* **2020**, *56*, 342. [CrossRef]
18. Smulter, N.; Lingehall, H.C.; Gustafson, Y.; Olofsson, B.; Engström, K.G. Delirium after cardiac surgery: Incidence and risk factors. *Interact. Cardiovasc. Thorac. Surg.* **2013**, *17*, 790–796. [CrossRef]
19. Onuma, H.; Inose, H.; Yoshii, T.; Hirai, T.; Yuasa, M.; Kawabata, S.; Okawa, A. Preoperative risk factors for delirium in patients aged ≥75 years undergoing spinal surgery: A retrospective study. *J. Int. Med. Res.* **2020**, *48*, 300060520961212. [CrossRef]
20. Shin, H.J.; Choi, S.L.; Na, H.S. Prevalence of postoperative delirium with different combinations of intraoperative general anesthetic agents in patients undergoing cardiac surgery: A retrospective propensity-score-matched study. *Medicine* **2021**, *100*, e26992. [CrossRef]
21. Momeni, M.; Khalifa, C.; Lemaire, G.; Watremez, C.; Tircoveanu, R.; Van Dyck, M.; Kahn, D.; Martins, M.R.; Mastrobuoni, S.; De Kerchove, L.; et al. Propofol plus low-dose dexmedetomidine infusion and postoperative delirium in older patients undergoing cardiac surgery. *Br. J. Anaesth.* **2020**, *126*, 665–673. [CrossRef]
22. Galyfos, G.C.; Geropapas, G.E.; Sianou, A.; Sigala, F.; Filis, K. Risk factors for postoperative delirium in patients undergoing vascu-lar surgery. *J. Vasc. Surg.* **2017**, *66*, 937–946. [CrossRef]
23. Miyazaki, S.; Yoshitani, K.; Miura, N.; Irie, T.; Inatomi, Y.; Ohnishi, Y.; Kobayashi, J. Risk factors of stroke and delirium after off-pump coronary artery bypass surgery. *Interact. Cardiovasc. Thorac. Surg.* **2010**, *12*, 379–383. [CrossRef]
24. Thorsteinsdóttir, S.A.; Sveinsdóttir, H.; Snædal, J. Óráð eftir opna hjartaaðgerð: Kerfisbundin samantekt á algengi, áhættuthá-ttum og afleiðingum [Delirium after open cardiac surgery: systematic review of prevalence, risk factors and consequences]. *Laeknabladid* **2015**, *101*, 305–311.
25. Russell, M.D.; Pinkerton, C.; Sherman, K.A.; Ebert, T.J.; Pagel, P.S. Predisposing and Precipitating Factors Associated With Postoperative Delirium in Patients Undergoing Cardiac Surgery at a Veterans Affairs Medical Center: A Pilot Retrospective Analysis. *J. Cardiothorac. Vasc. Anesth.* **2020**, *34*, 2103–2110. [CrossRef]

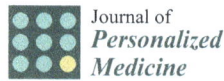 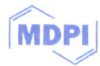

Article

A Descriptive Analysis of Hybrid Cannulated Extracorporeal Life Support

Sebastian D. Sahli [1], Alexander Kaserer [1,*], Julia Braun [2], Raed Aser [3], Donat R. Spahn [4,†] and Markus J. Wilhelm [3,†]

[1] Institute of Anesthesiology, University and University Hospital Zurich, 8091 Zurich, Switzerland; sebastian.sahli@usz.ch
[2] Epidemiology, Biostatistics and Prevention Institute, Departments of Epidemiology and Biostatistics, University of Zurich, 8057 Zurich, Switzerland; julia.braun@uzh.ch
[3] Clinic for Cardiac Surgery, University Heart Center, University and University Hospital Zurich, 8091 Zurich, Switzerland; raed.aser@usz.ch (R.A.); markus.wilhelm@usz.ch (M.J.W.)
[4] Formerly, Institute of Anesthesiology, University and University Hospital Zurich, 8091 Zurich, Switzerland; donat.spahn@swisspbm.ch
* Correspondence: alexander.kaserer@usz.ch; Tel.: +41-(0)43-254-07-81
† These authors contributed equally to this work.

Abstract: Background: Extracorporeal life support (ECLS) is pivotal for sustaining the function of failing hearts and lungs, and its utilization has risen. In cases where conventional cannulation strategies prove ineffective for providing adequate ECLS support, the implementation of an enhanced system with a third cannula may become necessary. Hybrid ECLS may be warranted in situations characterized by severe hypoxemia of the upper extremity, left ventricular congestion, and dilatation. Additionally, it may also be considered for patients requiring respiratory support or experiencing hemodynamic instability. Method: All hybrid ECLS cases of adults at the University Hospital Zurich, Switzerland, between January 2007 and December 2019 with initial triple cannulation were included. Data were collected via a retrospective review of patient records and direct export of the clinical information system. Results: 28 out of 903 ECLS cases were initially hybrid cannulated (3.1%). The median age was 57 (48.2 to 60.8) years, and the sex was equally distributed. The in-hospital mortality of hybrid ECLS was high (67.9%). In-hospital mortality rates differ depending on the indication (ARDS: 36.4%, refractory cardiogenic shock: 88.9%, cardiopulmonary resuscitation: 100%, post-cardiotomy: 100%, others: 75%). Survivors exhibited a lower SAPS II level compared with non-survivors (20.0 (12.0 to 65.0) vs. 55.0 (45.0 to 73.0)), and the allogenic transfusion of platelet concentrate was observed to be less frequent for survivors (0.0 (0.0) vs. 1.8 (2.5) units). Conclusion: The in-hospital mortality rate for hybrid ECLS was high. Different indications showed varying mortality rates, with survivors having lower SAPS II scores and requiring fewer platelet concentrate transfusions. These findings highlight the complexities of hybrid ECLS outcomes in different clinical scenarios and underline the importance of rigorous patient selection.

Keywords: extracorporeal circulation; ECMO; ECLS; mortality; outcome

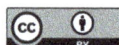

1. Introduction

Extracorporeal life support (ECLS) plays a critical role in cardiopulmonary assistance once conventional measures have been exhausted. It has become a key support instrument during organ recovery or the onset of destination therapy [1,2]. Veno-venous (V-V) and veno-arterial (VA) ECLS modifications are standard. If oxygenation or ventilation is predominantly impaired, support is provided by passing venous blood through an artificial lung membrane. The afferent limb returns the decarboxylated and oxygenated blood back to the venous system. If a patient has cardiovascular disease and consequent hemodynamic instability, the blood from the membrane lung can be returned to the arterial system. In addition to oxygenation, it provides a pumping function to maintain perfusion pressure. Specific limitations such as age, malignancy, or patient preference, as well as structural and staffing requirements, must be considered [3].

During ECLS therapy, the supply of oxygenated blood to the coronary arteries and brain is dependent on pulmonary function (V-V) or retrograde aortic flow (VA) [4]. However, a modified system with an additional third (sometimes even fourth) cannula is required in some cases in which ineffective ECLS support presents with a mixed picture of hypoperfusion and hypoxemia due to competing or insufficient circuits [5]. Unfortunately, only few data are available on the adaption of the ECLS toward a hybrid cannulation [6–12]. According to the Extracorporeal Life Support Organization (ELSO) report 2017, 2% of adults supported with ECLS for cardiac failure and less than 1% on ECMO for respiratory failure are managed with a hybrid cannulation [13]. The analysis of the Chinese Extracorporeal Life Support Registry (CSECLS) showed 19 (0.6%) initial hybrid configurations out of 3102 adult ECLS cases between 2017 and 2019 [6].

In recent years, there has been increasing awareness of the need for a standardized nomenclature for ECLS therapy. The use of standardized descriptions of the ECLS modification allows for comparison and analysis (also from center to center). For this purpose, the ELSO position papers provide concrete rules for the ECLS nomenclature [14,15]. The use of a hyphen to differentiate drainage cannulas to the left of the hyphen from return cannulas to the right of the hyphen is the core of any cannulation abbreviation. The hyphen itself symbolizes the membrane lung (ML). According to the Maastricht Treaty for ECLS nomenclature [14], the third added cannula is defined by an additional capital letter placed outside the existing cannulas. For example, if a second venous drain cannula is added, the letter "V" is placed to the left of the hyphen and outside the first drain cannula, resulting in "VV-A". In a V-A setup, if an additional re-entry cannula is inserted alongside the initial arterial cannula to improve systemic oxygenation, the letter "V" is added to the outer right to indicate post-ML flow (return): "V-AV". The insertion of an arterial cannula into a "V-V" configuration is indicated as "V-VA". Consequently, the order of configurations during ECLS therapy reflects the patient's temporal support needs and conveys a chronological sequence. But the nomenclature lacks differentiation between V-V and V-A proportional support. And from a physiological standpoint, V-VA is indistinguishable from V-AV. Besides the cannula hierarchy and localization, the position of the cannula tip and its dimensions are also relevant.

The hybrid ECLS configuration supports patients with combined cardiopulmonary failure who cannot be successfully assisted with the conventional veno-venous or veno-arterial alone. Hybrid ECLS may be required in conditions of severe hypoxemia of the upper extremity, also known as Harlequin syndrome or north–south syndrome [2], but also in cases of left ventricular congestion and dilatation [5]. A supplemental inflow cannula can be placed in the internal jugular vein to deliver oxygenated blood to the pulmonary circulation. This helps correct differential hypoxemia by directing oxygenated blood back to the right ventricle then through the pulmonary circulation, left ventricle, and out to the coronary arteries and aortic arch vessels [16]. Another relevant indication includes ECMO patients receiving respiratory support who also exhibit concurrent hemodynamic instability, particularly in cases of right heart failure [5] but also in left or biventricular failure. For hemodynamic support, an arterial perfusion cannula is inserted into the circuit, usually via the femoral or subclavian artery.

This study investigates the factors that determine the association between hybrid ECLS and patient outcomes. We analyzed all initially hybrid cannulated ECLS cases between the period from 2007 to 2019 at the University Hospital of Zurich.

2. Materials and Methods

2.1. Study Design

All hybrid ECLS cases of adults at the University Hospital Zurich (USZ) in Switzerland between January 2007 and December 2019 with initial triple cannulation were included.

We differentiated V-AV (efferent limb venous; afferent arteriovenous) and VV-A (efferent limb veno-venous; afferent arterial) configuration. Modifications at a later stage of V-A ECLS and V-V ECMO were not included. Further exclusion criteria were age below 18 years and documented refusal of general consent. We grouped indications for hybrid ECLS therapy into five common categories according to the current literature [1,2,6,8]: "acute respiratory distress syndrome", "refractory cardiogenic shock", "cardiopulmonary resuscitation", "post-cardiotomy", and "other".

The study was approved, and the requirement for written informed consent was waived by the Cantonal Ethics Commission of Zurich, Switzerland (BASEC-Nr. 2019-01926).

2.2. Assessment of Hybrid Modification

Based on the underlying disease, the indication was for either V-V or V-A ECLS therapy. In cases where the medical team, consisting of a cardiac anesthesiologist or intensivist, a cardiac surgeon, and a perfusionist, identified inadequate drainage or perfusion during initialization of the baseline configuration, a hybrid procedure was adapted. As recommended in the ELSO nomenclature, when a VVA mode configuration is implemented primarily for cardiac support, it is expressed as V-AV (initial indication V-A).

2.3. Study Endpoints

We recorded the in-hospital mortality to compare survivors and non-survivors. Furthermore, 1-year mortality was assessed.

2.4. Data Collection and Variables

Data were collected via a retrospective review of the medical records of all included patients with hybrid ECLS (medical history, last laboratory values, ECLS configuration and duration, complications, length of ICU stay, and outcomes) and direct export of the clinical information system via medical controlling (age, gender, number of transfused red blood cells, fresh frozen plasma, and platelet concentrate, and length of hospital stay).

2.5. Statistical Analysis

For descriptive statistics, we show the median and interquartile range (IQR 25% to 75%) for continuous variables. For categorical variables, we show counts (n) and proportions (%). Due to the small sample size, we chose not to present statistical tests, as this would quickly lead to a multiple-testing problem, which in turn would make any meaningful statistical interpretation impossible.

3. Results

We screened 903 ECLS cases between 2007 and 2019, 28 of whom (3.1%) were instances of initial hybrid ECLS cannulation and matched the inclusion criteria (Figure 1).

3.1. Patient Characteristics and Mortality

The median age was 57 (48.2 to 60.8) years, and the sex was equally distributed. The most frequent comorbidity at the time of ECLS cannulation was coronary artery disease (17.9%). Patients had a high SAPS II within the first 24 h of ICU admission, and survivors exhibited a lower SAPS II level compared with non-survivors (20.0 (12.0 to 65.0) vs. 55.0 (45.0 to 73.0)) (Table 1). Fifteen patients died during hybrid ECLS therapy, and four patients died after weaning. Overall, the in-hospital mortality was high (19 out of 28, 67.9%) (Table 2).

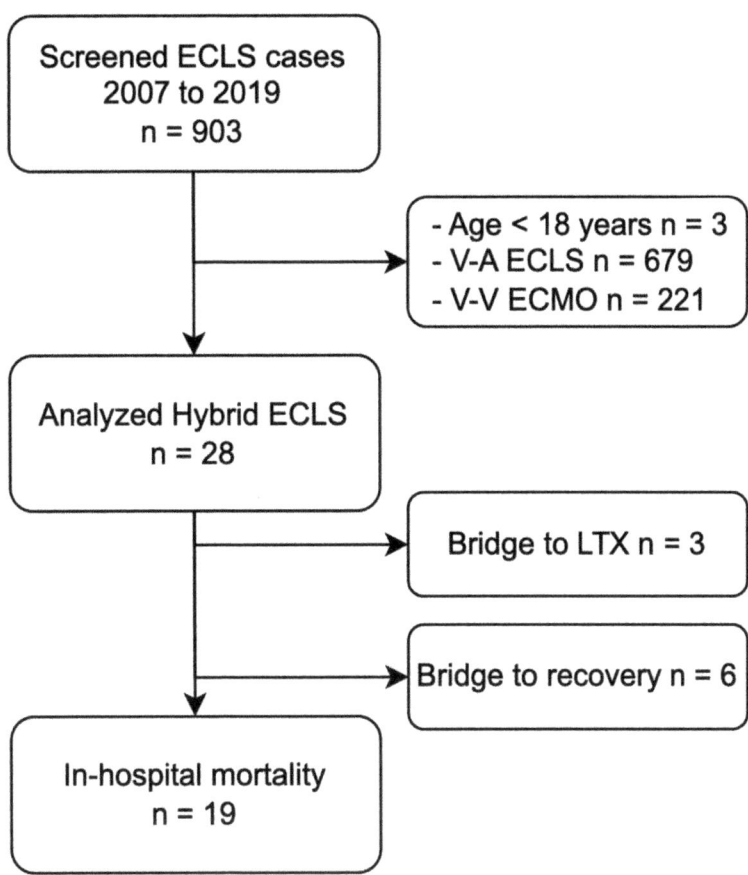

Figure 1. Flowchart of patient selection and hybrid ECLS outcome. Abbreviations: ECLS, extracorporeal life support; ECMO, extracorporeal membrane oxygenation; LTX, lung transplantation; V-A, veno-arterial; V-V, veno-venous.

Table 1. Characteristics of hybrid ECLS patients stratified for survivors and non-survivors.

	All [n = 28]	Survivors [n = 9]	Non-Survivors [n = 19]
Patient characteristics			
Age (years)	57.0 (48.2 to 60.8)	55.0 (32.0 to 57.5)	57.0 (49.0 to 64.0)
BMI (kg/m^2)	25.5 (22.7 to 33.0)	30.1 (22.1 to 36.2)	24.7 (22.5 to 31.2)
Sex (female)	14 (50.0)	4 (44.4)	10 (52.6)
SAPS II (points)	53.5 (29.3 to 68.0)	20.0 (12.0 to 65.0)	55.0 (45.0 to 73.0)
Charlson comorbidity index	2.5 (1.0 to 3.8)	2.0 (1.0 to 3.5)	3.0 (1.0 to 4.0)
Comorbidities			
Coronary artery disease	5 (17.9)	1 (11.1)	4 (21.1)
Congestive heart failure	3 (10.7)	0 (0.0)	3 (15.8)
Peripheral vascular disease	2 (7.1)	0 (0.0)	2 (10.5)
Obstructive pulmonary disease	3 (10.7)	0 (0.0)	3 (15.8)
Diabetes mellitus	3 (10.7)	0 (0.0)	3 (15.8)
Chronic kidney disease	0 (0.0)	0 (0.0)	0 (0.0)

Table 1. Cont.

	All [n = 28]	Survivors [n = 9]	Non-Survivors [n = 19]
Baseline laboratory parameters			
pH	7.273 (7.140 to 7.455) (7)	7.273 (7.121 to 7.392)	7.282 (7.132 to 7.458)
pO_2 (kPa)	7.9 (7.1 to 12.1) (7)	8.1 (7.1 to 22.7)	7.9 (6.9 to 12.1)
pCO_2 (kPa)	5.8 (4.6 to 8.6) (7)	7.7 (5.7 to 12.9)	5.6 (4.4 to 8.4)
Lactate (mmol/L)	2.5 (1.5 to 6.9) (7)	1.6 (1.2 to 4.4)	2.9 (1.5 to 10.1)
Hemoglobin (g/L)	89.5 (79.3 to 102.5) (0)	86.0 (77.0 to 102.0)	92.0 (80.0 to 112.0)
Myoglobin (µg/L)	164.0 (58.0 to 536.0) (5)	175.0 (101.3 to 334.3)	164.0 (48.0 to 859.0)
Creatinine (µmol/L)	115.0 (78.0 to 171.0) (1)	109.0 (73.5 to 142.0)	127.0 (78.3 to 196.5)

Data presented as median and interquartile range (IQR). Categorical variables as number and percentage (%). If necessary, missing data are indicated in parentheses [n]. Abbreviations: BMI, body mass index; ECLS, extracorporeal life support; SAPS II, simplified acute physiology score II.

Table 2. Description of hybrid ECLS cases stratified for survivors and non-survivors.

	All [n = 28]	Survivors [n = 9]	Non-Survivors [n = 19]
ECLS			
Indication			
ARDS	11 (39.3)	7 (77.8)	4 (21.1)
Refractory cardiogenic shock	9 (32.1)	1 (11.1)	8 (42.1)
Cardiopulmonary resuscitation	2 (7.1)	0 (0.0)	2 (10.5)
Post-cardiotomy	2 (7.1)	0 (0.0)	2 (10.5)
Other	4 (14.3)	1 (11.1)	3 (15.8)
ECLS outcome			
Successful weaning	9 (32.1)	6 (66.7)	3 (15.8)
Bridge to assist device	1 (3.6)	0 (0.0)	1 (5.3)
Bridge to lung transplantation	3 (10.7)	3 (33.3)	0 (0.0)
Complications During ECLS Therapy			
Transfusions			
Red blood cells (units)	4.0 (2.0 to 7.8) / 6.8 (9.0)	4.0 (2.5 to 6.5) / 8.3 (13.1)	4.0 (1.0 to 8.0) / 6.0 (6.5)
Fresh frozen plasma (units)	0.0 (0.0 to 1.0) / 0.6 (1.0)	0.0 (0.0 to 1.0) / 0.3 (0.5)	0.0 (0.0 to 1.0) / 0.7 (1.2)
Platelet concentrate (units)	0.0 (0.0 to 2.0) / 1.3 (2.2)	0.0 (0.0 to 0.0) / 0.0 (0.0)	1.0 (0.0 to 3.0) / 1.8 (2.5)
Major bleeding	8 (28.6)	2 (22.2)	6 (31.6)
Intracranial bleeding	1 (3.6)	0 (0.0)	1 (5.3)
Stroke	0 (0.0)	0 (0.0)	0 (0.0)
Liver failure	1 (3.6)	1 (11.1)	0 (0.0)
Renal replacement therapy	12 (42.9)	4 (44.4)	8 (42.1)
Ischemia extremities	3 (10.7)	1 (11.1)	2 (10.5)
Open chest therapy	4 (14.3)	0 (0.0)	4 (21.1)
Duration			
Length ECLS (days)	8.5 (3.3 to 14.3)	11.0 (8.0 to 18.5)	6.0 (2.0 to 12.0)
Length ICU (days)	19.5 (8.5 to 31.3)	26.0 (18.5 to 42.0)	13.0 (6.0 to 29.0)
Length of hospital stay (days)	26.5 (8.5 to 43.0)	32.0 (19.5 to 82.0)	23.0 (6.0 to 34.0)
Mortality			
In-hospital mortality	19 (67.9)	0 (0.0)	19 (100)
Death during ECLS therapy	15 (53.6)	0 (0.0)	15 (78.9)
1-year survival	7 (26.9) (2)	7 (77.8)	0 (0.0)

Data presented as median and interquartile range (IQR). For transfusion counts, mean and standard deviation (SD) are listed as well. Categorical variables as number and percentage (%). If necessary, missing data are indicated in parentheses [n]. Abbreviations: ARDS, acute respiratory distress syndrome; ECLS, extracorporeal life support; ICU, intensive care unit.

3.2. Outcomes of Survivors

Six patients were successfully weaned, and three patients had bridged-to-lung transplantation. Except for two patients who were lost to follow-up, all patients were alive at one year (Table 3).

Table 3. Outcome of survivors.

Patient	ECLS	Outcome	Discharge	1-y Survival
1	V-AV	Successful weaning	Transfer to another hospital	Loss of follow-up
2	V-AV	Successful weaning	Rehabilitation	Yes
3	VV-A	Successful weaning	Transfer to another hospital	Yes
4	VV-A	Successful weaning	At home	Yes
5	VV-A	Successful weaning	Rehabilitation	Yes
6	VV-A	Bridge to LTX	At home	Yes
7	VV-A	Bridge to LTX	Rehabilitation	Yes
8	V-AV	Successful weaning	At home	Loss of follow-up
9	V-AV	Bridge to LTX	At home	Yes

Abbreviations: 1-y Survival, 1-year survival; ECLS, extracorporeal life support; LTX, lung transplantation; VV-A, ECLS mode venovenous-arterial; V-AV, ECLS mode veno-venoarterial.

3.3. Hybrid ECLS Indication

The largest group of hybrid ECLS indications was represented by patients suffering from ARDS who showed a higher survival at hospital discharge (7 out of 11 cases), resulting in an in-hospital mortality of 36.4% (Figure 2). Patients with refractory cardiogenic shock showed a high in-hospital mortality of 88.9% (eight out of nine). Patients with hybrid ECLS indications for cardiopulmonary resuscitation and post-cardiotomy showed 100% in-hospital mortality (two out of two each). The indication "other" consisted of two patients suffering from acute respiratory insufficiency (not defined as ARDS), one patient with pulmonary scleroderma, and one patient diagnosed with obstructive shock due to an atrial tumor. Only one of the four patients in the "other" group survived, resulting in an in-hospital mortality of 75%.

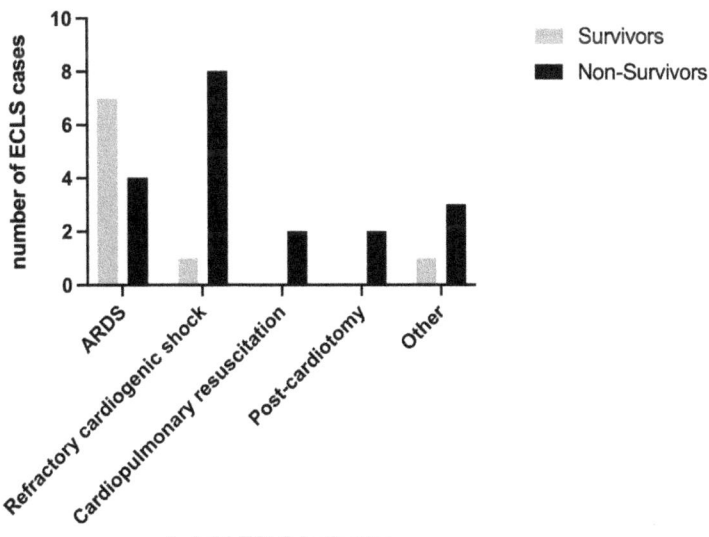

Figure 2. Survivors and non-survivors stratified by indication of hybrid ECLS.

3.4. Hybrid ECLS Cannulation Details

Most cannulations were performed peripherally using the Seldinger technique (71.4%). Six ECLS cases were performed as V-AV configurations and the others as VV-A (Figure 3). Regarding the efferent ECLS limb, a venous femoral drain was installed in each case. The further combinations of V-AV and VV-A modifications are shown in Figure 4. The in-hospital mortality was higher in the VV-A group (17 of 22, 77.3%) compared to the V-AV group (2 of 6, 33.3%).

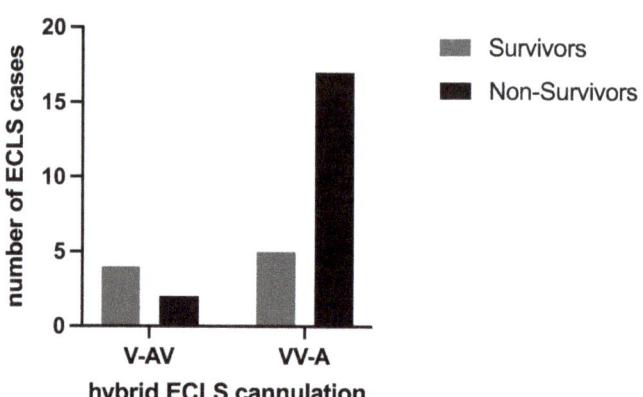

Figure 3. Survivors and non-survivors stratified by cannulation of hybrid ECLS.

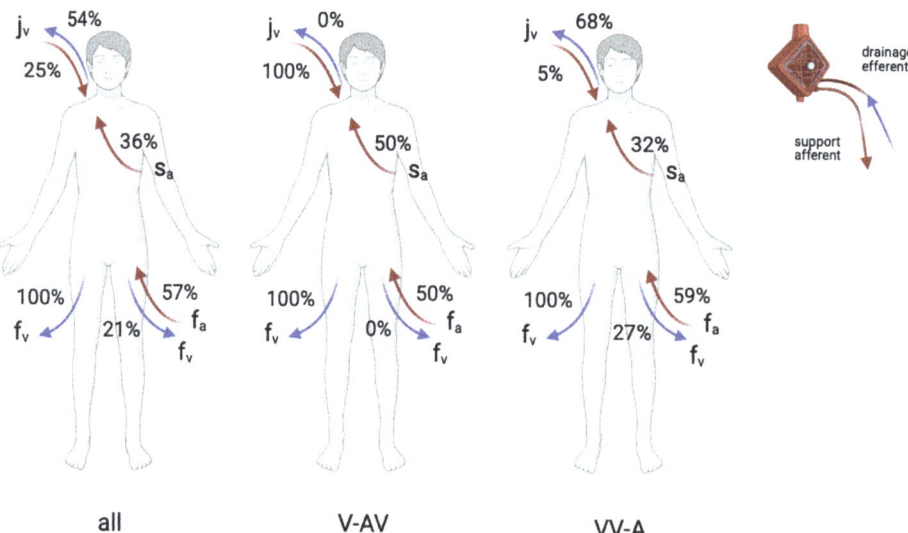

Figure 4. Cannulation sites for hybrid configuration according to frequency. (All) All hybrid ECLS cannulation percentages together, (V-AV) venous-arteriovenous hybrid modification (6 cases), and (VV-A) venovenous-arterial hybrid modification (22 cases). The cannulation site of one case (efferent right atrium and afferent pulmonary artery, 3.6% each) is not shown due to visibility. The right or left site is arbitrary. Note that the sum of percentages is equal to 300% due to three cannulation sites each. Abbreviations: j_v internal jugular vein; s_a subclavian artery; f_v femoral vein; f_a femoral artery. Created with BioRender.com, accessed on 9 December 2023, with confirmation of publication and licensing rights.

3.5. Hybrid ECLS Complications

The allogenic transfusion of platelet concentrate was higher for non-survivors compared to survivors (1.8 vs. 0 units). Besides renal replacement therapy, major bleeding events were the most frequent complications and were also observed more frequently in the cohort of non-survivors (Table 2).

4. Discussion

This retrospective single-center study reports 28 initially hybrid-cannulated ECLS cases at the University Hospital of Zurich in the period from 2007 to 2019. We observed a high in-hospital mortality of 67.9% (n = 19); 4 of the 19 non-survivors died after ECLS weaning. The most frequent diagnosis at the time of hybrid ECLS installation was ARDS (11 patients), with more survivors than non-survivors in this group. Overall, non-survivors had a higher SAPS II and more frequently received transfusion of allogenic platelet concentrates.

Although only a few studies are available for hybrid ECLS with a low number of included patients (3 to 26 patients) [6–12,17], the in-hospital mortality observed at our institution is in line with that in recently published studies. Biscotti et al. [9] and Ius et al. [11] reported lower mortality rates of 57.1% and 50.0%, but they also included patients who were initially conventionally cannulated and only later modified to a hybrid strategy. ECLS indications in those studies were predominantly pulmonary diseases. Looking separately at the indication ARDS of our study, the in-hospital mortality is as low as 36.4%. This is in accordance with a study published in 2010 with a small number of cases [12]. A recently published retrospective study of patients with predominant ARDS on V-V ECMO support requiring a change to V-VA support showed an in-hospital mortality rate of 37% [18].

We recently published our outcome analysis of 679 V-A [19] and 221 V-V [20] ECLS cases. The frequency of hybrid ECLS in our institution (3%) is in line with published data of ELSO [13] (2% of adults supported for cardiac failure and less than 1% for respiratory failure). The Chinese Extracorporeal Life Support Registry (CSECLS) states that 0.6% of initial hybrid configurations between 2017 and 2019 [6].

The institutional comparison shows a higher in-hospital mortality rate between conventionally V-A-assisted and hybrid-assisted ECLS cases (V-A vs. hybrid: indication post-cardiotomy 70.7% vs. 100%, cardiopulmonary resuscitation 67.9% vs. 100%, refractory cardiogenic shock 47.0% vs. 88.9%). Mortality is nearly identical between V-V and hybrid-assisted patients (V-V vs. hybrid: indication ARDS 36.2% vs. 36.4%). It is likely that the sicker patients needed more support initially. In terms of selection bias, the initial hybrid cannulated patients also have a higher mortality rate. This finding should certainly be taken into account when the treatment team is considering hybrid cannulation. As compared to V-A and hybrid cannulation, V-V cannulated cases have fewer major bleeding complications (16.7%, 25.2%, and 28.6%) or leg ischemias (6.3%, 13.4%, and 10.7%) at our institution. Complication rates are similar between V-A and hybrid. But the small number of hybrid cannulated cases must be considered.

In our study, we describe three patients who were treated with a hybrid ECLS bridging procedure and who were finally treated with a lung transplantation. Bridging to heart transplantation was not observed. It is crucial to note that ECLS therapy is not a definitive treatment but rather a bridge to recovery in the context of significant lung or heart failure, as well as a bridge to decision-making. ECLS often necessitates high doses of anticoagulation, posing a risk of bleeding, particularly intracranial, and requiring massive transfusion [21]. This is associated with adverse effects on patient morbidity and mortality [22], not to mention the additional immunologic effects and increased risk of a positive cross-match in planned transplants. On the positive side, advancements in treatment protocols and expertise in specialized centers over the past decade have made bridging to lung transplantation feasible for patients with end-stage lung disease, yielding reasonable outcomes [23]. Apart from optimized gas exchange, these patients experience reduced sedation requirements and less confinement to the hospital bed, allowing for better-organized physiotherapy and nutrition. While pharmacological treatments for end-stage heart failure have improved, the majority of patients succumb to the disease, with heart transplantation being the sole option [24]. However, the scarcity of donor organs has led to the establishment of ECLS as the primary alternative, serving as a bridge to recovery or as a bridge-to-bridge, allowing for the subsequent implantation of a long-term device, or as a bridge-to-transplant [25]. It is important to recognize ECLS as a high-risk procedure with significant morbidity and mortality. Additionally, the limited availability of healthcare resources and ethical considerations must be taken into account.

The cannulation strategy depends on the underlying pathology and is implemented in various ways. Nevertheless, principles are now emerging to improve systemic oxygenation or cardiac unloading [26,27]. A V-VA configuration has been proposed in patients with differential hypoxia (Harlequin syndrome) or secondary heart failure (e. g., right ventricular impairment) after V-V ECMO initiation [5]. We describe six cases with an in-hospital mortality of 33.3%. The other cannulation mode, VV-A, combines the need for higher venous drainage with the possibility of providing both circulatory and respiratory support and is more complex [5]. Interestingly, this cannulation strategy is predominant in our study. Their markedly higher in-hospital mortality of 77.3% reflects this statement.

Besides renal replacement therapy, major bleeding events were the most prevalent complication during hybrid ECLS therapy. With a frequency of 28.6%, major bleeding occurred less frequently than described in the literature, with almost every second patient suffering from major bleeding [8]. In contrast to our expectation, complications like leg ischemia and intracranial bleeding were rare in our cohort. Werner et al. [7] and Mihu et al. [8] reported higher incidences of these complications, despite a conservative anticoagulation regimen. As a possible reason, they mention that more than half of their patients were externally cannulated and that there was no radiological imaging of the brain prior to initiation of ECLS. A patient-oriented balance needs to be struck between the postulated benefits of hybrid cannulation and the potential harm it may cause. There is an increased risk of bleeding, infection, and thrombosis. Additional technical problems arise, such as the difficulty of flow measurement with parallel systems, as well as their flow regulation.

Retrograde aortic flow may lead to impaired myocardial function and pulmonary congestion as an inherent disadvantage of VA treatment. In addition to hybrid cannulation, another strategy to improve hemodynamics in cardiogenic shock is venting [28]. The first systematic review of left ventricular unloading with Impella in addition to VA-ECMO ("ECMELLA") described an improved survival and neurological outcome despite higher complication rates compared to VA-ECMO alone [29].

5. Conclusions

The in-hospital mortality rate for hybrid ECLS was high. Different indications showed varying mortality rates, with survivors having lower SAPS II scores and requiring fewer platelet concentrate transfusions. These findings highlight the complexities of hybrid ECLS outcomes in different clinical scenarios and underline the need for rigorous patient selection.

6. Limitations

The small sample size of the study presents challenges in generalizing the results. Results from a single high-volume ECMO center may have limited applicability to broader populations. In addition, the inclusion of patients over an extended period of time includes the potential for changes in both the patient population and standards of care that may have evolved over time. Finally, the analysis focuses on a heterogeneous cohort, reflecting the inherent complexity of this specialized therapy. Despite these limitations, retrospective studies provide valuable insights into associations between variables and serve as a basis for generating hypotheses that merit further investigation.

Author Contributions: Conceptualization, S.D.S., A.K., D.R.S. and M.J.W.; formal analysis, S.D.S. and J.B.; data curation, S.D.S.; writing—original draft preparation, S.D.S.; writing—review and editing, S.D.S., A.K., J.B., R.A., D.R.S. and M.J.W.; visualization, S.D.S.; supervision, A.K.; project administration, S.D.S. All authors have read and agreed to the published version of the manuscript.

Funding: This research received no external funding.

Institutional Review Board Statement: The study was conducted in accordance with the Declaration of Helsinki. The study was reviewed, and the requirement for written informed consent was waived by the Cantonal Ethics Commission of Zurich, Switzerland (BASEC No. 2019-01926).

Informed Consent Statement: The study was reviewed by the Cantonal Ethics Commission of Zurich, Switzerland. Patients with documented refused informed consent were excluded.

Data Availability Statement: The data are not publicly available due to privacy or ethical restrictions.

Conflicts of Interest: S.D.S., J.B., R.A. and M.J.W. have no conflicts of interest to declare. A.K. has received support from Bayer AG (Switzerland) and CSL Behring GmbH (Switzerland) for lecturing. D.R.S.'s former academic department receives grant support from the Swiss National Science Foundation, Berne, Switzerland, the Swiss Society of Anesthesiology and Perioperative Medicine (SSAPM), Berne, Switzerland; the Swiss Foundation for Anesthesia Research, Zurich, Switzerland; and CSL Vifor (International) AG, St. Gallen, Switzerland. D.R.S. is co-chair of the ABC-Trauma Faculty, sponsored by unrestricted educational grants from Alexion Pharma Germany GmbH, Munich, Germany; CSL Behring GmbH, Marburg, Germany; and LFB Biomédicaments, Courtaboeuf Cedex, France. D.R.S. received honoraria/travel support for consulting or lecturing from Alliance Rouge, Bern, Switzerland; Danube University of Krems, Austria; European Society of Anesthesiology and Intensive Care, Brussels, BE; International Foundation for Patient Blood Management, Basel, Switzerland; Korean Society of Anesthesiologists, Seoul, Korea; Network for the Advancement of Patient Blood Management, Haemostasis and Thrombosis, Paris, France; Society for the Advancement of Blood Management, Mount Royal NJ, Alexion Pharmaceuticals Inc., Boston, MA; AstraZeneca AG, Baar, Switzerland; Bayer AG, Zürich, Switzerland; B. Braun Melsungen AG, Melsungen, Germany; Baxter AG, Glattpark, Switzerland; CSL Behring GmbH, Hattersheim am Main, Germany and Berne, Switzerland; CSL Vifor (Switzerland) Villars-sur-Glâne, Switzerland; CSL Vifor (International), St. Gallen, Switzerland; Celgene International II Sàrl, Couvet, Switzerland; Daiichi Sankyo AG, Thalwil, Switzerland; Haemonetics, Braintree, MA, USA; iSEP, Nantes, France, LFB Biomédicaments, Courtaboeuf Cedex, France; Merck Sharp & Dohme, Kenilworth, New Jersey, USA; Novo Nordisk Health Care AG, Zurich, Switzerland; Octapharma AG, Lachen, Switzerland; Pharmacosmos A/S, Holbaek, Denmark; Pierre Fabre Pharma, Alschwil, Switzerland; Portola Schweiz GmbH, Aarau, Switzerland; Roche Diagnostics International Ltd., Reinach, Switzerland; Sarstedt AG & Co., Sevelen, Switzerland, and Nümbrecht, Germany; Shire Switzerland GmbH, Zug, Switzerland; Takeda, Glattpark, Switzerland; Werfen, Bedford, MA; and Zuellig Pharma Holdings, Singapore, Singapore.

References

1. Brodie, D.; Slutsky, A.S.; Combes, A. Extracorporeal Life Support for Adults with Respiratory Failure and Related Indications: A Review. *JAMA* **2019**, *322*, 557–568. [CrossRef] [PubMed]
2. Guglin, M.; Zucker, M.J.; Bazan, V.M.; Bozkurt, B.; El Banayosy, A.; Estep, J.D.; Gurley, J.; Nelson, K.; Malyala, R.; Panjrath, G.S.; et al. Venoarterial ECMO for Adults: JACC Scientific Expert Panel. *J. Am. Coll. Cardiol.* **2019**, *73*, 698–716. [CrossRef] [PubMed]
3. Assmann, A.; Beckmann, A.; Schmid, C.; Werdan, K.; Michels, G.; Miera, O.; Schmidt, F.; Klotz, S.; Starck, C.; Pilarczyk, K.; et al. Use of extracorporeal circulation (ECLS/ECMO) for cardiac and circulatory failure -A clinical practice Guideline Level 3. *ESC Heart Fail* **2022**, *9*, 506–518. [CrossRef] [PubMed]
4. Frenckner, B.; Broman, M.; Broomé, M. Position of draining venous cannula in extracorporeal membrane oxygenation for respiratory and respiratory/circulatory support in adult patients. *Crit. Care* **2018**, *22*, 163. [CrossRef] [PubMed]
5. Brasseur, A.; Scolletta, S.; Lorusso, R.; Taccone, F.S. Hybrid extracorporeal membrane oxygenation. *J. Thorac. Dis.* **2018**, *10*, S707–S715. [CrossRef] [PubMed]
6. Li, C.; Xie, H.; Li, J.; Qin, B.; Lu, J.; Zhang, J.; Lv, L.; Li, B.; Zhou, C.; Yin, Y.; et al. Dynamic and Hybrid Configurations for Extracorporeal Membrane Oxygenation: An Analysis of the Chinese Extracorporeal Life Support Registry. *ASAIO J.* **2022**, *68*, 547–552. [CrossRef]
7. Werner, N.L.; Coughlin, M.; Cooley, E.; Haft, J.W.; Hirschl, R.B.; Bartlett, R.H.; Mychaliska, G.B. The University of Michigan Experience with Veno-Venoarterial Hybrid Mode of Extracorporeal Membrane Oxygenation. *ASAIO J.* **2016**, *62*, 578–583. [CrossRef]

8. Mihu, M.R.; Mageka, D.; Swant, L.V.; El Banayosy, A.; Maybauer, M.O.; Harper, M.D.; Koerner, M.M.; El Banayosy, A. Veno-arteriovenous extracorporeal membrane oxygenation-A single center experience. *Artif. Organs.* **2021**, *45*, 1554–1561. [CrossRef]
9. Biscotti, M.; Lee, A.; Basner, R.C.; Agerstrand, C.; Abrams, D.; Brodie, D.; Bacchetta, M. Hybrid configurations via percutaneous access for extracorporeal membrane oxygenation: A single-center experience. *ASAIO J.* **2014**, *60*, 635–642. [CrossRef]
10. Cakici, M.; Gumus, F.; Ozcinar, E.; Baran, C.; Bermede, O.; Inan, M.B.; Durdu, M.S.; Sirlak, M.; Akar, A.R. Controlled flow diversion in hybrid venoarterial-venous extracorporeal membrane oxygenation. *Interact. Cardiovasc. Thorac. Surg.* **2018**, *26*, 112–118. [CrossRef]
11. Ius, F.; Sommer, W.; Tudorache, I.; Avsar, M.; Siemeni, T.; Salman, J.; Puntigam, J.; Optenhoefel, J.; Greer, M.; Welte, T.; et al. Veno-veno-arterial extracorporeal membrane oxygenation for respiratory failure with severe haemodynamic impairment: Technique and early outcomes. *Interact. Cardiovasc. Thorac. Surg.* **2015**, *20*, 761–767. [CrossRef]
12. Stöhr, F.; Emmert, M.Y.; Lachat, M.L.; Stocker, R.; Maggiorini, M.; Falk, V.; Wilhelm, M.J. Extracorporeal membrane oxygenation for acute respiratory distress syndrome: Is the configuration mode an important predictor for the outcome? *Interact. Cardiovasc. Thorac. Surg.* **2011**, *12*, 676–680. [CrossRef]
13. Thiagarajan, R.R.; Barbaro, R.P.; Rycus, P.T.; McMullan, D.M.; Conrad, S.A.; Fortenberry, J.D.; Paden, M.L. Extracorporeal Life Support Organization Registry International Report 2016. *ASAIO J.* **2017**, *63*, 60–67. [CrossRef] [PubMed]
14. Broman, L.M.; Taccone, F.S.; Lorusso, R.; Malfertheiner, M.V.; Pappalardo, F.; Di Nardo, M.; Belliato, M.; Bembea, M.M.; Barbaro, R.P.; Diaz, R.; et al. The ELSO Maastricht Treaty for ECLS Nomenclature: Abbreviations for cannulation configuration in extracorporeal life support—A position paper of the Extracorporeal Life Support Organization. *Crit. Care* **2019**, *23*, 36. [CrossRef]
15. Conrad, S.A.; Broman, L.M.; Taccone, F.S.; Lorusso, R.; Malfertheiner, M.V.; Pappalardo, F.; Di Nardo, M.; Belliato, M.; Grazioli, L.; Barbaro, R.P.; et al. The Extracorporeal Life Support Organization Maastricht Treaty for Nomenclature in Extracorporeal Life Support. A Position Paper of the Extracorporeal Life Support Organization. *Am. J. Respir. Crit. Care Med.* **2018**, *198*, 447–451. [CrossRef] [PubMed]
16. Sorokin, V.; MacLaren, G.; Vidanapathirana, P.C.; Delnoij, T.; Lorusso, R. Choosing the appropriate configuration and cannulation strategies for extracorporeal membrane oxygenation: The potential dynamic process of organ support and importance of hybrid modes. *Eur. J. Heart Fail.* **2017**, *19* (Suppl. S2), 75–83. [CrossRef] [PubMed]
17. Kukielski, C.; Jarrett Davis, C.; Saberi, A.; Chaudhary, S. Veno-arteriovenous (V-AV) ECMO configuration: A single-center experience. *J. Card. Surg.* **2022**, *37*, 1254–1261. [CrossRef] [PubMed]
18. Erlebach, R.; Wild, L.C.; Seeliger, B.; Rath, A.K.; Andermatt, R.; Hofmaenner, D.A.; Schewe, J.C.; Ganter, C.C.; Müller, M.; Putensen, C.; et al. Outcomes of patients with acute respiratory failure on veno-venous extracorporeal membrane oxygenation requiring additional circulatory support by veno-venoarterial extracorporeal membrane oxygenation. *Front. Med.* **2022**, *9*, 1000084. [CrossRef]
19. Sahli, S.D.; Kaserer, A.; Braun, J.; Halbe, M.; Dahlem, Y.; Spahn, M.A.; Rössler, J.; Krüger, B.; Maisano, F.; Spahn, D.R.; et al. Predictors associated with mortality of extracorporeal life support therapy for acute heart failure: Single-center experience with 679 patients. *J. Thorac. Dis.* **2022**, *14*, 1960–1971. [CrossRef]
20. Neumann, E.; Sahli, S.D.; Kaserer, A.; Braun, J.; Spahn, M.A.; Aser, R.; Spahn, D.R.; Wilhelm, M.J. Predictors associated with mortality of veno-venous extracorporeal membrane oxygenation therapy. *J. Thorac. Dis.* **2023**, *15*, 2389–2401. [CrossRef]
21. Javidfar, J.; Bacchetta, M. Bridge to lung transplantation with extracorporeal membrane oxygenation support. *Curr. Opin. Organ. Transpl.* **2012**, *17*, 496–502. [CrossRef] [PubMed]
22. Spahn, D.R.; Muñoz, M.; Klein, A.A.; Levy, J.H.; Zacharowski, K. Patient Blood Management: Effectiveness and Future Potential. *Anesthesiology* **2020**, *133*, 212–222. [CrossRef] [PubMed]
23. Tipograf, Y.; Salna, M.; Minko, E.; Grogan, E.L.; Agerstrand, C.; Sonett, J.; Brodie, D.; Bacchetta, M. Outcomes of Extracorporeal Membrane Oxygenation as a Bridge to Lung Transplantation. *Ann. Thorac. Surg.* **2019**, *107*, 1456–1463. [CrossRef] [PubMed]
24. Combes, A. Mechanical circulatory support for end-stage heart failure. *Metabolism* **2017**, *69*, S30–S35. [CrossRef] [PubMed]
25. Hansen, B.; Singer Englar, T.; Cole, R.; Catarino, P.; Chang, D.; Czer, L.; Emerson, D.; Geft, D.; Kobashigawa, J.; Megna, D.; et al. Extracorporeal membrane oxygenation as a bridge to durable mechanical circulatory support or heart transplantation. *Int. J. Artif. Organs.* **2022**, *45*, 604–614. [CrossRef] [PubMed]
26. Shah, A.; Dave, S.; Goerlich, C.E.; Kaczorowski, D.J. Hybrid and parallel extracorporeal membrane oxygenation circuits. *JTCVS Tech.* **2021**, *8*, 77–85. [CrossRef]
27. Napp, L.C.; Kühn, C.; Hoeper, M.M.; Vogel-Claussen, J.; Haverich, A.; Schäfer, A.; Bauersachs, J. Cannulation strategies for percutaneous extracorporeal membrane oxygenation in adults. *Clin. Res. Cardiol. Off. J. Ger. Card. Soc.* **2016**, *105*, 283–296. [CrossRef]

28. Lüsebrink, E.; Orban, M.; Kupka, D.; Scherer, C.; Hagl, C.; Zimmer, S.; Luedike, P.; Thiele, H.; Westermann, D.; Massberg, S.; et al. Prevention and treatment of pulmonary congestion in patients undergoing venoarterial extracorporeal membrane oxygenation for cardiogenic shock. *Eur. Heart J.* **2020**, *41*, 3753–3761. [CrossRef]
29. Thevathasan, T.; Füreder, L.; Fechtner, M.; Mørk, S.R.; Schrage, B.; Westermann, D.; Linde, L.; Gregers, E.; Andreasen, J.B.; Gaisendrees, C.; et al. Left-Ventricular Unloading with Impella During Refractory Cardiac Arrest Treated with Extracorporeal Cardiopulmonary Resuscitation: A Systematic Review and Meta-Analysis. *Crit. Care Med.* **2024**. *online ahead of print*. [CrossRef]

Disclaimer/Publisher's Note: The statements, opinions and data contained in all publications are solely those of the individual author(s) and contributor(s) and not of MDPI and/or the editor(s). MDPI and/or the editor(s) disclaim responsibility for any injury to people or property resulting from any ideas, methods, instructions or products referred to in the content.

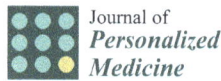

Article

Depression and Anxiety in Heart Transplant Recipients: Prevalence and Impact on Post-Transplant Outcomes

Emyal Alyaydin [1,*], Juergen Reinhard Sindermann [1], Jeanette Köppe [2], Joachim Gerss [2], Patrik Dröge [3], Thomas Ruhnke [3], Christian Günster [3], Holger Reinecke [1] and Jannik Feld [2]

[1] Department of Cardiology I—Coronary and Peripheral Vascular Disease, Heart Failure, University Hospital Muenster, Albert Schweitzer Campus 1, A1, 48149 Muenster, Germany
[2] Institute of Biostatistics and Clinical Research, University of Muenster, 48149 Muenster, Germany
[3] AOK Research Institute (WIdO), 10178 Berlin, Germany
* Correspondence: e.alyaydin@gmx.de; Tel.: +49-(0)-251-83-43-201

Abstract: Background: Depression and anxiety (DA) are common mental disorders in patients with chronic diseases, but the research regarding their prevalence in heart transplantation (HTx) is still limited. Methods: We performed an analysis of the prevalence and prognostic relevance of DA in patients who underwent HTx between 2010 and 2018 in Germany. Data were obtained from Allgemeine Ortskrankenkasse (AOK), which is the largest public health insurance provider. Results: Overall, 694 patients were identified. More than a third of them were diagnosed with DA before undergoing HTx (n = 260, 37.5%). Patients with DA more often had an ischaemic cardiomyopathy ($p < 0.001$) and a history of previous myocardial infarction ($p = 0.001$) or stroke ($p = 0.002$). The prevalence of hypertension ($p < 0.001$), diabetes ($p = 0.004$), dyslipidaemia ($p < 0.001$) and chronic kidney disease ($p = 0.003$) was higher amongst transplant recipients with DA. Patients with DA were more likely to suffer an ischaemic stroke ($p < 0.001$) or haemorrhagic stroke ($p = 0.032$), or develop septicaemia ($p = 0.050$) during hospitalisation for HTx. Our analysis found no significant differences between the groups with respect to in-hospital mortality. The female sex and mechanical circulatory support were associated with an inferior prognosis. Pretransplant non-ischaemic cardiomyopathy was related to a favourable outcome. Conclusions: DA affect up to a third of the population undergoing HTx, with a greater prevalence in patients with comorbidities. DA are associated with a higher incidence of stroke and septicaemia after HTx.

Keywords: depression; anxiety; orthotopic heart transplantation; in-hospital mortality; survival

1. Introduction

Depression and anxiety (DA) are protean disorders with a wide range of symptom severity and an increasing prevalence worldwide. According to recent reports, each condition alone affects approximately 4% of the global population [1]. DA prevalence is much higher in patients suffering from chronic diseases [2]. To date, studies indicate that roughly one-fifth of the patients diagnosed with heart failure (HF) also exhibit DA. This disease combination has been linked to an overall poor prognosis and lower quality of life (QoL) [3,4]. Nevertheless, patients with advanced HF who are awaiting heart transplantation (HTx) have to carry an even greater emotional burden, resulting in frequent recurrences and more severe symptoms of DA. Thus, it is to be expected that DA prevalence is higher in patients undergoing orthotopic HTx. In addition to a poor QoL, DA have been associated with limited compliance to recommended treatments and behaviours. All these factors may have deleterious consequences for the graft function in transplantation. A previous retrospective single-centre analysis reported an increased rate of hospitalisations and infectious complications after HTx in patients with DA [5]. The cardiovascular side effects of antidepressants are another factor limiting the treatment alternatives in most cases to selective serotonin reuptake inhibitors (SSRIs) only. Thus, the guidelines for the care of heart transplant recipients recommend regular evaluation of the mental health of patients undergoing HTx [6].

The aim of our study was to assess the prevalence and prognostic relevance of DA in patients undergoing orthotopic HTx.

2. Materials and Methods

2.1. Data Retrieval

Our study comprises data on adult heart transplant recipients anonymously retrieved from Allgemeine Ortskrankenkasse (AOK), which is an alliance of eleven regional funds covering up to a third of the population in Germany. According to recent reports, AOK provided insurance coverage for 25.938.841 affiliated persons and family members in the year 2018. In contrast to the private sector, public health insurance in Germany does not depend on gross income, health status, region, profession or age.

The timeline of our analysis was based on the index hospitalisation for orthotopic heart transplantation (HTx) (operation and procedure code 5-375.0). The study population was preselected among all subjects hospitalised for heart failure, coronary artery disease, myocardial infarction, peripheral artery disease, stroke and patients who underwent coronary or peripheral artery interventions in either an ambulant or stationary setting between 2008 and 2018.

The study included 694 adult patients who were insured by AOK and underwent HTx between 1 January 2010 and 31 December 2018. Baseline patient comorbidities were assessed using data from the two years that preceded the index hospitalisation. Follow-up data were collected until 31 December 2019. The median (interquartile range (IQR)) follow-up was 5.9 (IQR: 5.0) years. The information retrieved included primary, secondary and tertiary care results that were analysed in a coded manner. Diagnoses were documented according to the 10th Revision of the German Modification of International Classification of Diseases (ICD-10-GM). The diagnostic and therapeutic procedures performed were encoded using the German Modification of the Operation and Procedure Classification System (OPS). Anatomical Therapeutic Chemical codes (ATC-codes) were used for the prescribed medical treatment.

Data sampling was approved by the Ethics Committee of the Landesaerztekammer Westfalen-Lippe and the Medical Faculty of the University of Muenster (2019-212-f-S).

2.2. Patient Population

We initially identified 852 patients who were hospitalised for orthotopic HTx (OPS: 5-375.0) between 1 January 2010 and 31 December 2018. Of these, 39 patients were excluded because they were <18 years of age at the time of the HTx procedure. In addition, 119 patients were excluded because of incomplete data. The study population was stratified into two groups according to whether a diagnosis of depression or anxiety was made prior to HTx (ICD-10-GM-Code: F30–F39 and F41) or not. We did not have access to detailed information regarding the methods implemented for the psychological assessment of the patients.

The primary outcome of our analyses was in-hospital mortality. The secondary endpoints included major adverse cardiovascular events, new onset or relapse of DA during the period covered by the study, and overall survival. Since, in most cases, both depression and anxiety are present simultaneously, and notably, most of the patients with depression have concurrent anxiety, we considered these conditions as a composite entity [1].

2.3. Statistics

The assessment of the impact of DA on the outcome of patients who had undergone HTx was performed using binary multivariable logistic regression models, which comprised major comorbidities and cardiovascular risk factors. Odds ratios with unadjusted 95% confidence intervals (CIs) for all features are shown in the graphs. Survival analyses were conducted using Kaplan–Meier estimators. Medication rates 90 days after index hospitalisation were estimated using competing risk models by calculating the cumulative incidence, where death was considered as a competing risk.

Quantitative data are reported as medians (IQRs) and compared using a two-sided Wilcoxon test. Qualitative data are presented as absolute values (percentages) and were compared using a two-sided chi-squared test.

All p-values of the test procedures described above are purely descriptive and unadjusted. Inferential statistics are intended to be exploratory (hypotheses-generating), not confirmatory, and are interpreted accordingly.

Statistical analyses were performed using R version 4.0.2.

3. Results

3.1. Patient Characteristics

A total of 694 patients who underwent HTx from 2010 to 2018, the period covered by our study, were evaluated. More than a third of this population had documented diagnoses of DA prior to HTx (n = 260, 37.5%). We observed no statistically noticeable intergroup disparities in age, sex or previous mechanical circulatory support (MCS). Whilst the prevalence of cerebrovascular (CVD) and peripheral arterial disease (PAD) did not differ between the two groups, antecedent cardiac disease of ischaemic origin was more frequent amongst those diagnosed with DA (n = 276, 63.6% vs. n = 200, 76.9%; p < 0.001). Additionally, patients assigned to the DA group were more likely to have had a previous myocardial infarction (n = 129, 29.7% vs. n = 108, 41.5%; p = 0.001), percutaneous coronary interventions (n = 54, 12.4% vs. n = 51, 19.6%; p = 0.011) or stroke (n = 54, 12.4% vs. n = 55, 21.2%; p = 0.002). A closer look at the evaluable cardiovascular risk factors (CVRFs) and comorbidities revealed differences in the prevalence of hypertension (n = 356, 82.0% vs. n = 237, 91.2%; p < 0.001), diabetes (n = 144, 33.2% vs. n = 115, 44.2%), dyslipidaemia (n = 290, 66.8% vs. n = 207, 79.6%; p < 0.001) and chronic kidney disease (n = 288, 66.4% vs. n = 200, 76.9%; p = 0.003). Furthermore, patients with DA were more often smokers (n = 95, 21.9% vs. n = 88, 33.8%; p < 0.001). We found no differences in the use of cardiovascular medications, including betablockers, statins, platelet aggregation inhibitors (PAIs); and oral anticoagulants on baseline assessment (Table 1).

Table 1. Baseline characteristics.

Characteristics	Non-DA n = 434	DA n = 260	Study Population n = 694	p-Value
Female, n (%)	90 (20.7)	64 (24.6)	154 (22.2)	0.234
Male, n (%)	344 (79.3)	196 (75.4)	540 (77.8)	0.234
VAD, n (%)	105 (24.2)	70 (26.9)	175 (25.2)	0.423
Age, median (IQR)	52.52 (14.53)	54.28 (11.70)	53.12 (13.56)	0.053
Previous acute myocarditis, n (%)	56 (12.9)	34 (13.1)	90 (13.0)	0.947
Dilated cardiomyopathy, n (%)	325 (74.9)	195 (75.0)	520 (74.9)	0.973
Non-dilated cardiomyopathy, n (%)	44 (10.1)	23 (8.8)	67 (9.7)	0.577
Ischaemic heart disease, n (%)	276 (63.6)	200 (76.9)	476 (68.6)	<0.001
Hypertension, n (%)	356 (82.0)	237 (91.2)	593 (85.4)	<0.001
Diabetes, n (%)	144 (33.2)	115 (44.2)	259 (37.3)	0.004
Dyslipidaemia, n (%)	290 (66.8)	207 (79.6)	497 (71.6)	<0.001
Obesity, n (%)	127 (29.3)	86 (33.1)	213 (30.7)	0.292
Smoking, n (%)	95 (21.9)	88 (33.8)	183 (26.4)	<0.001
Atrial flutter/fibrillation, n (%)	297 (68.4)	177 (68.1)	474 (68.3)	0.922
PAD, n (%)	30 (6.9)	23 (8.8)	53 (7.6)	0.353
CVD, n (%)	40 (9.2)	26 (10.0)	66 (9.5)	0.733
Chronic kidney disease, n (%)	288 (66.4)	200 (76.9)	488 (70.3)	0.003
Cancer, n (%)	44 (10.1)	24 (9.2)	68 (9.8)	0.697
No previous listing, n (%)	187 (43.1)	82 (31.5)	269 (38.8)	0.003
Previous MI, n (%)	129 (29.7)	108 (41.5)	237 (34.1)	0.001

Table 1. Cont.

Characteristics	Non-DA n = 434	DA n = 260	Study Population n = 694	p-Value
Previous PCI, n (%)	54 (12.4)	51 (19.6)	105 (15.1)	0.011
Previous stroke, n (%)	54 (12.4)	55 (21.1)	109 (15.7)	0.002
PAIs, n (%)	51 (11.8)	34 (13.1)	85 (12.2)	0.606
OACs, n (%)	106 (24.4)	65 (25.0)	171 (24.6)	0.865
PAIs in combination with OACs, n (%)	44 (10.1)	26 (10.0)	70 (10.1)	0.953
ACE-Is/AT1-antagonists, n (%)	204 (47.0)	126 (48.5)	330 (47.6)	0.710
Statins, n (%)	109 (25.1)	67 (25.8)	176 (25.4)	0.848
Betablockers, n (%)	252 (58.1)	153 (58.8)	405 (58.4)	0.840

Data are presented as number (percentage) or median (IQR). DA—depression and anxiety, VAD—ventricular assist device, PAD—peripheral artery disease, CVD—cerebrovascular disease, PCI—percutaneous coronary intervention, MI—myocardial infarction, PAIs—platelet aggregation inhibitors, OACs—oral anticoagulants, ACE-Is—angiotensin-converting enzyme inhibitors, AT1-antagonists—angiotensin 1 receptor antagonists.

3.2. In-Hospital Treatment

We observed no differences between the groups concerning the frequency of MCS, the duration of ventilatory support, the incidence of acute HF or renal failure, the frequency of renal replacement therapy, bleeding episodes, or the need for the supplementary transfusion of blood products. However, patients in the DA group developed ischaemic stroke (n = 27, 6.2% vs. n = 37, 14.2% in DA; $p < 0.001$), haemorrhagic stroke (n = 10, 2.3% vs. n = 14, 5.4% in DA; $p = 0.032$) and septicaemia (n = 65, 15.0% vs. n = 54, 20.8%; $p = 0.050$) more frequently than their unaffected counterparts. During index hospitalisation, 59 (22.7%) patients with a previous history of DA experienced a relapse of depression, whereas new depression was documented in only 26 cases. Similarly, 29 (11.2%) patients from the DA group had a recurrence of anxiety, but the prevalence of new anxiety was much lower. The data were censored due to confidentiality regulations (Table 2).

Table 2. Outcome.

Characteristics	Non-DA n = 434	DA n = 260	Overall Population n = 694	p-Value
ECMO, n (%)	65 (15.0)	34 (13.1)	99 (14.3)	0.488
Acute renal failure, n (%)	184 (42.4)	107 (41.2)	291 (41.9)	0.748
Renal replacement therapy, n (%)	287 (66.1)	173 (66.5)	460 (66.3)	0.912
Death (discharge status), n (%)	62 (14.3)	42 (16.2)	104 (15.0)	0.505
Ischaemic stroke, n (%)	27 (6.2)	37 (14.2)	64 (9.2)	<0.001
Haemorrhagic stroke, n (%)	10 (2.3)	14 (5.4)	24 (3.5)	0.032
Bleeding, n (%)	172 (39.6)	106 (40.8)	278 (40.1)	0.767
Ventilation, median (IQR)	71 (279)	66 (306)	70 (289)	0.933
Hospitalisation, median (IQR)	129 (130.3)	137 (142.8)	133 (137.0)	0.511
In-hospital CPR, n (%)	63 (14.5)	33 (12.7)	96 (13.8)	0.501
Blood transfusion, n (%)	393 (90.6)	234 (90.0)	627 (90.3)	0.811
Septicaemia, n (%)	65 (15.0)	54 (20.8)	119 (17.1)	0.050
Allograft rejection, n (%)	88 (20.3)	58 (22.3)	146 (21.0)	0.525
New depression, n (%)	26 (6.0)	N/A	26 (3.7)	N/A
Depression relapse, n (%)	N/A	59 (22.7)	59 (8.5)	N/A
New anxiety, n (%)	<10	N/A	N/A	N/A
Anxiety relapse, n (%)	N/A	29 (11.2)	29 (4.2)	N/A
PAIs	36 (10.0)	25 (11.9)	61 (10.7)	0.478
OACs, n (%)	<10	<10	N/A	0.740
PAIs in combination with OACs, n (%)	<10	<10	N/A	0.190
ACE-Is/AT-blockers, n (%)	41 (11.4)	27 (12.9)	68 (11.9)	0.602
Statins, n (%)	59 (16.4)	46 (21.9)	105 (18.4)	0.101
Betablockers, n (%)	14 (3.9)	15 (7.1)	29 (5.1)	0.088

Data are presented as number (percentage) or median (IQR). DA—depression and anxiety, ECMO—extracorporeal membrane oxygenation, PAIs—platelet aggregation inhibitors, OACs—oral anticoagulants, ACE-Is—angiotensin-converting enzyme inhibitors, AT1-antagonists—angiotensin 1 receptor antagonists. N/A—not applicable.

3.3. Outcome

We observed no significant differences between the two study groups with respect to the primary outcome measure (Table 2). The five-year survival rates were 65.7% and 73.1% in the groups with and without a diagnosis of DA before HTx, respectively (Figure 1).

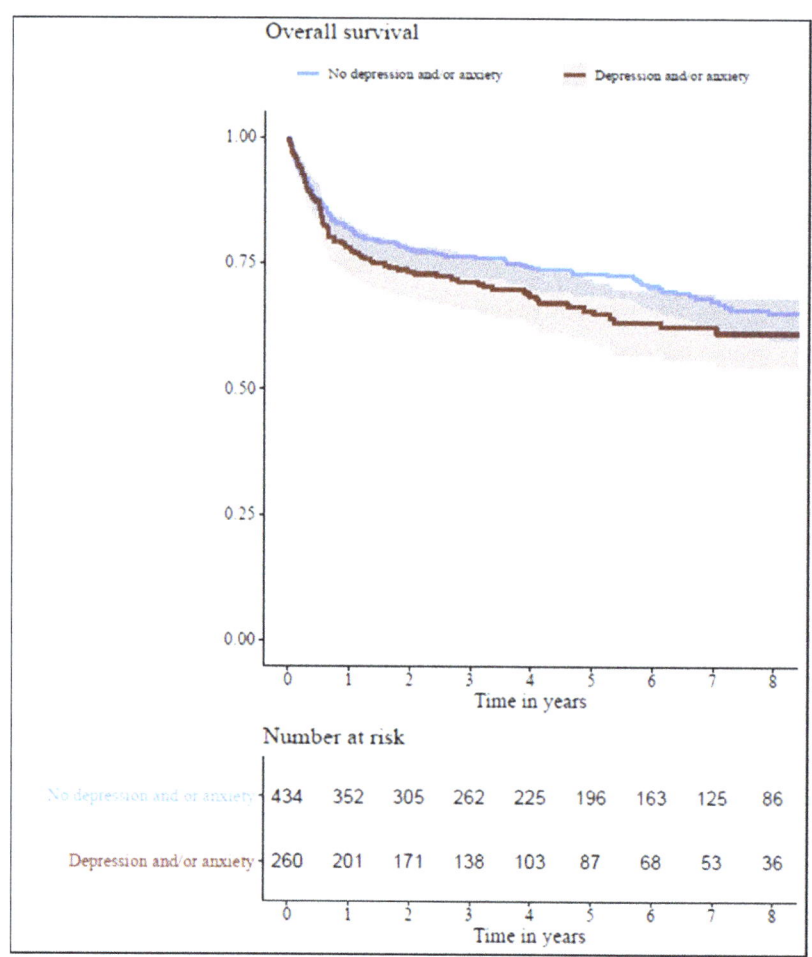

Figure 1. Kaplan–Meier survival estimates. Comparison of the overall survival in patients with DA (red line) and without DA (blue line) in long-term follow-up. DA—depression and anxiety.

However, our findings revealed that the female sex and use of extracorporeal membrane oxygenation (ECMO) during index hospitalisation were associated with inferior outcomes in a multivariate logistic regression analysis. By contrast, non-ischaemic cardiomyopathy was a determinant related to a prognostic advantage after HTx (Figure 2).

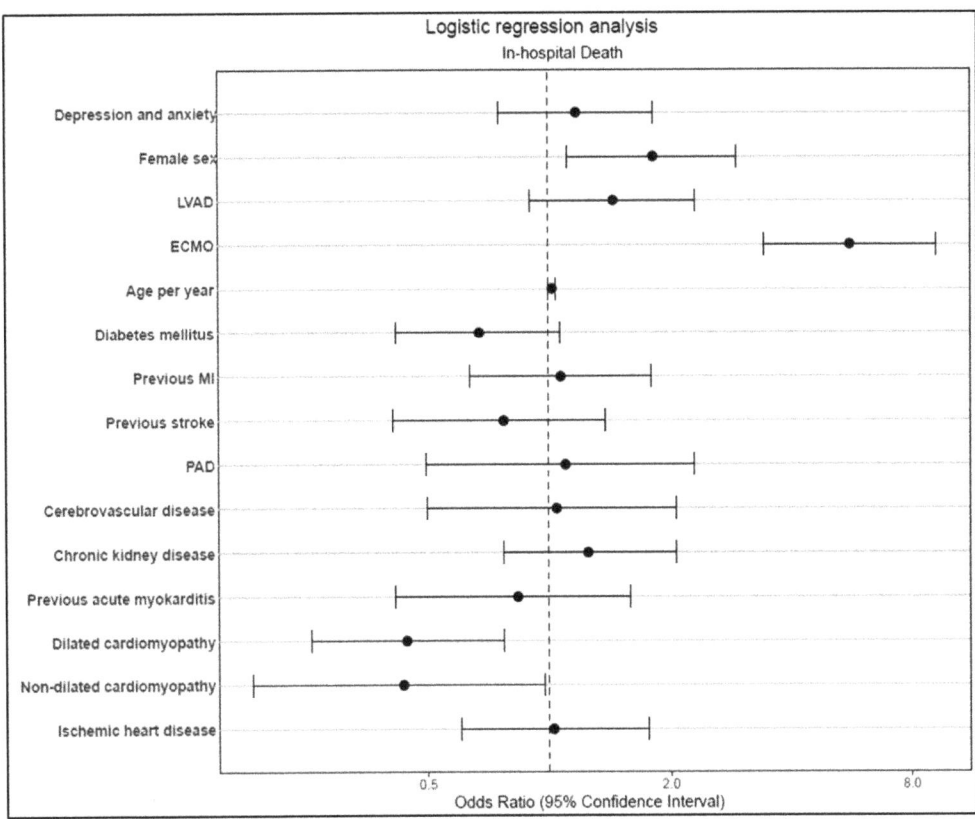

Figure 2. In-hospital mortality during index hospitalisation for heart transplantation. LVAD—left ventricular assist device, ECMO—extracorporeal membrane oxygenation, MI—myocardial infarction, PAD—peripheral artery disease.

4. Discussion

To the best of our knowledge, this is the first study to examine the impact of DA on the outcome of HTx recipients in a relatively large patient cohort.

Approximately one-third of the patients enrolled in our study were diagnosed with DA before HTx, which is more than previously reported [5]. One possible explanation for the increased prevalence of these disorders may relate to the modality of data acquisition. Both disorders were considered for our analyses as a composite entity. We recognise that the overall prevalence of DA cannot be calculated as a simple sum of the included diagnoses because patients often present with an overlap between the two conditions. Additionally, the ICD-10-GM system includes a range of disease severities, which allows us to reflect not only major DA episodes, but also milder cases.

Women are generally underrepresented amongst HTx recipients, and they constituted approximately one-fifth of the overall population of our cohort [7]. These results may reflect the lack of awareness of heart disease in women due to their beneficial cardiovascular profile, resulting in a presentation at an older age with advanced disease and comorbidity profiles. Additionally, as previously reported, the prevalence of DA was higher amongst women (41.6%) in our study population compared to men (36.3%) [1]. However, regardless of sex, the disease burden by far exceeded the magnitude in the general population.

4.1. Pretransplant Diagnoses and CVRF

The prevalence of DA was higher in patients with typical cardiovascular morbidity profiles, including diabetes, hypertension, dyslipidaemia and chronic kidney disease. Previous studies have reported a bidirectional relationship between chronic diseases and mental health [2,8]. DA can add to the burden of physical illnesses, as an unhealthy lifestyle and non-adherence to prescribed medications may further accelerate the progression of the underlying conditions [9,10]. In contrast, the perception of physical illness and related concerns are associated with a higher DA prevalence [11]. Interestingly, the risk of developing mental health problems has been reported to differ based on specific patterns of physical morbidity. Thus, there are discrepancies when determining the risk of developing DA even amongst patients with cardiometabolic and cardio/cerebrovascular profiles [8]. Additionally, although active tobacco smoking during the previous six months is considered a relative contraindication for HTx, the prevalence of smoking was 11% higher amongst patients with DA in the two years preceding HTx [12]. The evidence in this field supports the notion that the risk of becoming a smoker and the daily amount of smoking is higher in people with DA, whereas the likelihood of quitting is lower than in the general population [13,14]. This may be due to the reciprocal relationship between daily habits and mental health, as smoking is usually associated with a higher risk of developing depression in addition to the bidirectional relationship between the diseases of the body and mind [15].

The higher rate of ischaemic heart disease (IHD), myocardial infarction and stroke amongst HTx recipients with DA may also be a consequence of this population's higher cardiovascular risk profile. Previous reports have defined numerous physiologic links between DA and IHD, including dysregulation of the autonomic nervous system and peripheral vascular function, increased sympathetic tone, inflammatory activity, elevated heart rate, and endothelial dysfunction [16]. Similarly, although the overall prevalence of DA in patients with HF is higher than in the general population, differences between non-ischaemic cardiomyopathy and IHD have been reported. Particularly, patients hospitalised for acute myocardial infarction are considered to be at a high risk for major DA [17].

Although the burden of DA in patients with cancer is generally considered to be higher than in other diseases, we observed no differences in the prevalence of malignancies between the study groups [18]. This may be a consequence of the preselection of the patients, as the current recommendations for being added to the HTx waiting list take into account disease curability and require additional remission time, dependent on the type of cancer, before patients are considered for transplantation. Similarly, symptomatic CVD, PAD and severe obesity are relative contraindications for HTx [12]. This may result in a preselection of patients free from disease or only milder cases.

The prevalence of DA increases along with a prolonged time on the HTx waiting list [19]. This may explain the higher rate of previous listings in the DA group. In a world with an increasing prevalence of HF and a shortage of donor organs, awaiting HTx will be associated with a prolonged waiting time and an increased likelihood of death, which can further augment the burden on the patients' mental health. Thus, closer monitoring and interdisciplinary assessment while being listed for HTx are required.

4.2. In-Hospital Treatment

The incidence of ischaemic or haemorrhagic stroke following HTx was higher in patients with DA, despite a comparable rate of prescription of anticoagulants and PAIs. However, it is critical to recognise that antidepressants and SSRIs in particular, which are widely prescribed for patients with DA and HF because of their limited cardiovascular side effects, can cause major bleeding and ischaemic events [20,21]. Possible explanations for the increased bleeding rate are their fibrinolytic properties and potential to reduce platelet adhesion. On the contrary, ischaemic events are linked to additional factors, including limited physical activity [22]. Caution is required when prescribing SSRIs with anticoagulants, as this may result in an augmented bleeding risk. A similar association was observed in antiplatelet therapy, where SSRI prescription was previously reported to increase the risk of bleeding by 42% when prescribed in addition to aspirin and by 57% in patients on a dual antiplatelet therapy [23,24]. It is essential to investigate the association between the use of SSRIs and bleeding in the population of patients undergoing HTx. Unfortunately, we did not have access to data regarding psychotropic medication use from the patients. Due to the modality of our study, we had permission to analyse only data related to the use of cardiac drugs and anticoagulants.

Results from antecedent research indicated an increased prevalence of infectious complications and septicaemia in patients with DA who were undergoing HTx [5]. On the one hand, these findings may be linked to inflammation, but on the other hand, the downregulation of the immune system in chronic DA may also contribute to the disease course [25]. As our report focuses on in-hospital treatment and outcomes, no direct relation between these findings and a sedentary lifestyle or fidelity to taking the prescribed medication can be suspected.

4.3. Relapse or Post-Transplant DA

Interestingly, a previous history of DA was associated with a greater risk for relapse during index hospitalisation. By contrast, the incidence of new DA was much lower. This evidence indicates the need for a thorough pretransplant assessment so that the medical team will be aware of the patient's condition after HTx.

4.4. Outcome

The five-year survival rate of the overall population was 70.4%, which is comparable with results to date [26]. Patients with DA had a slightly higher immediate post-transplant mortality, but it was not statistically significant. This can be due to the modality of our analyses, as we reported on in-hospital treatment and mortality in the immediate post-transplant period, whereas DA are more likely to have a long-term impact on a patient's QoL. The favourable prognosis in non-ischaemic cardiomyopathy may be due to the comorbidity profile of the patients. IHD was previously reported to be associated with a significantly inferior outcome in short- and long-term follow-up [27].

The female sex and ECMO support during index hospitalisation were both associated with a significantly inferior prognosis. We should note that the current available data on sex differences and outcomes after HTx are contradictory. According to recent registry reports, female patients have a superior overall survival than men [28]. Observational studies in smaller cohorts have indicated that many other related factors such as graft size and sex mismatch may be the factors influencing the patient's prognosis [29]. Due to the modality of our analyses, we cannot take into account these determinants.

ECMO therapy during index hospitalisation was also a factor associated with an inferior prognosis. We cannot differentiate between pre- or post-transplant short-term MCS, which limits the value of the findings. Additionally, there were no differences in the length of hospital stay between the groups, which may rule out persisting hemodynamic instability due to sustained graft failure [30,31].

4.5. Strengths and Limitations

One drawback of our study is its retrospective design and the use of administrative data, which can carry a risk of a selection bias or potential confounding factors outside the scope of our analyses. The retrieved data provide an opportunity to conduct analyses focused on outcome and major complications in large cohorts. Additionally, the use of ICD codes makes it possible to cover a range of disease severities and to reflect not only major DA episodes, but also milder cases. However, to reduce potential bias, the study findings still need to be investigated in a randomised manner.

Another drawback of this approach is the limited insight into the patients' clinical condition aside from the diagnoses. We report on the recovery rate, but we cannot take into account the grade of recovery (exercise capacity and NYHA class) after HTx. Additionally, some factors such as size and sex mismatch, donors' characteristics and recipients' laboratory results, which may influence the outcome of the patients, cannot be assessed.

5. Conclusions

DA are commonly diagnosed in patients undergoing HTx, particularly in those with multiple comorbidities. This underscores the bidirectional association between the disease of the body and the mind. Whilst we observed a higher prevalence of ischaemic stroke, haemorrhagic stroke and septicaemia in the immediate post-transplant period in patients diagnosed with DA, the latter had no prognostic relevance in long-term follow-up. Additionally, the incidence of new DA was lower than the rate of relapse in patients already diagnosed with these conditions. This observation suggests that pretransplant DA may set the stage for recurrent mental health disorders following HTx. Therefore, closer monitoring of these patients during the post-transplant phase is crucial to the success of the treatment mission.

Supplementary Materials: The following supporting information can be downloaded at: https://www.mdpi.com/article/10.3390/jpm13050844/s1, Supplementary Tables S1 and S2: Diagnoses and procedural codes; Table S3: In-hospital mortality during index hospitalisation for heart transplantation.

Author Contributions: Conceptualisation, E.A. and H.R.; methodology, E.A., J.F. and H.R.; software, P.D., C.G. and T.R.; validation, J.F. and J.R.S.; formal analysis, J.F., J.G. and J.K.; investigation, E.A.; resources, E.A.; data curation, P.D., C.G. and T.R.; writing—original draft preparation, E.A. and J.F.; writing—review and editing, J.K., J.G., P.D., C.G., T.R., H.R. and J.R.S.; visualisation, J.F.; supervision, H.R. and J.R.S.; project administration, H.R.; funding acquisition, H.R. All authors have read and agreed to the published version of the manuscript.

Funding: This study is part of the GenderVasc project (Gender-specific real care situation of patients with arteriosclerotic cardiovascular diseases) funded by The Federal Joint Committee, Innovation Committee (G-BA, Innovationsfond, number 01VSF18051). GenderVasc is a project conducted in cooperation with the AOK Research Institute of the AOK (WIdO).

Institutional Review Board Statement: Data sampling was approved by the Ethics Committee of the Landesaerztekammer Westfalen-Lippe and the Medical Faculty of the University of Muenster (2019-212-f-S).

Informed Consent Statement: Patient consent was not needed as only anonymised administrative data were used for this analysis.

Data Availability Statement: The authors confirm that the data utilised in this study cannot be made available in the manuscript, in the Supplementary Files or in a public repository due to German data protection laws ('Bundesdatenschutzgesetz', BDSG). Therefore, they are stored on a secure drive in the AOK Research Institute (WIdO), to facilitate replication of the results. Generally, access to data of statutory health insurance funds for research purposes is possible only under the conditions defined in German Social Law (SGB V § 287). Requests for data access can be sent as a formal proposal specifying the recipient and purpose of the data transfer to the appropriate data protection agency. Access to the data used in this study can only be provided to external parties under the conditions of a cooperation contract with this research project and after written approval by the sickness fund. For assistance in obtaining access to the data, please contact wido@wido.bv.aok.de.

Conflicts of Interest: There are no conflicts of interests in relation to this manuscript.

References

1. Depression and Other Common Mental Disorders: Global Health Estimates. World Health Organization. 2017. Available online: http://www.who.int/mental_health/management/depression/prevalence_global_health_estimates/en (accessed on 21 March 2023).
2. Chapman, D.P.; Perry, G.S.; Strine, T.W. The vital link between chronic disease and depressive disorders. *Prev. Chronic Dis.* **2005**, *2*, A14. [PubMed]
3. Celano, C.M.; Villegas, A.C.; Albanese, A.M.; Gaggin, H.K.; Huffman, J.C. Depression and Anxiety in Heart Failure: A Review. *Harv. Rev. Psychiatry.* **2018**, *26*, 175–184. [CrossRef]
4. Rutledge, T.; Reis, V.A.; Linke, S.E.; Greenberg, B.H.; Mills, P.J. Depression in heart failure a meta-analytic review of prevalence, intervention effects, and associations with clinical outcomes. *J. Am. Coll. Cardiol.* **2006**, *48*, 1527–1537. [CrossRef] [PubMed]

5. Delibasic, M.; Mohamedali, B.; Dobrilovic, N.; Raman, J. Pre-transplant depression as a predictor of adherence and morbidities after orthotopic heart transplantation. *J. Cardiothorac. Surg.* **2017**, *12*, 62. [CrossRef]
6. Costanzo, M.R.; Dipchand, A.; Starling, R.; Anderson, A.; Chan, M.; Desai, S.; Fedson, S.; Fisher, P.; Gonzales-Stawinski, G.; Martinelli, L.; et al. The International Society of Heart and Lung Transplantation Guidelines for the care of heart transplant recipients. *J. Heart Lung Transplant.* **2010**, *29*, 914–956. [CrossRef]
7. García-Cosío, M.D.; González-Vilchez, F.; López-Vilella, R.; Barge-Caballero, E.; Gómez-Bueno, M.; Martínez-Selles, M.; Arizón, J.M.; Rangel Sousa, D.; González-Costello, J. Gender differences in heart transplantation: Twenty-five year trends in the nationwide Spanish heart transplant registry. *Clin. Transplant.* **2020**, *34*, e14096. [CrossRef] [PubMed]
8. Ronaldson, A.; Arias de la Torre, J.; Prina, M.; Armstrong, D.; Das-Munshi, J.; Hatch, S.; Stewart, R.; Hotopf, M.; Dregan, A. Associations between physical multimorbidity patterns and common mental health disorders in middle-aged adults: A prospective analysis using data from the UK Biobank. *Lancet Reg. Health Eur.* **2021**, *8*, 100149. [CrossRef] [PubMed]
9. Grenard, J.L.; Munjas, B.A.; Adams, J.L.; Suttorp, M.; Maglione, M.; McGlynn, E.A.; Gellad, W.F. Depression and medication adherence in the treatment of chronic diseases in the United States: A meta-analysis. *J. Gen. Intern. Med.* **2011**, *26*, 1175–1182. [CrossRef]
10. Hare, D.L.; Toukhsati, S.R.; Johansson, P.; Jaarsma, T. Depression and cardiovascular disease: A clinical review. *Eur. Heart J.* **2014**, *35*, 1365–1372. [CrossRef]
11. Health Quality Ontario. Screening and management of depression for adults with chronic diseases: An evidence-based analysis. *Ont. Health Technol. Assess Ser.* **2013**, *13*, 1–45.
12. Mehra, M.R.; Canter, C.E.; Hannan, M.M.; Semigran, M.J.; Uber, P.A.; Baran, D.A.; Danziger-Isakov, L.; Kirklin, J.K.; Kirk, R.; Kushwaha, S.S. The 2016 International Society for Heart Lung Transplantation listing criteria for heart transplantation: A 10-year update. *J. Heart Lung Transplant.* **2016**, *35*, 1–23. [CrossRef]
13. Fergusson, D.M.; Goodwin, R.D.; Horwood, L.J. Major depression and cigarette smoking: Results of a 21-year longitudinal study. *Psychol. Med.* **2003**, *33*, 1357–1367. [CrossRef]
14. Breslau, N.; Peterson, E.L.; Schultz, L.R.; Chilcoat, H.D.; Andreski, P. Major depression and stages of smoking. A longitudinal investigation. *Arch. Gen. Psychiatry* **1998**, *55*, 161–166. [CrossRef]
15. Flensborg-Madsen, T.; von Scholten, M.B.; Flachs, E.M.; Mortensen, E.L.; Prescott, E.; Tolstrup, J.S. Tobacco smoking as a risk factor for depression. A 26-year population-based follow-up study. *J. Psychiatr. Res.* **2011**, *45*, 143–149. [CrossRef]
16. Vaccarino, V.; Badimon, L.; Bremner, J.D.; Cenko, E.; Cubedo, J.; Dorobantu, M.; Duncker, D.J.; Koller, A.; Manfrini, O.; Milicic, D.; et al. Depression and coronary heart disease: 2018 position paper of the ESC working group on coronary pathophysiology and microcirculation. *Eur. Heart J.* **2020**, *41*, 1687–1696. [CrossRef]
17. Lichtman, J.H.; Bigger, J.T.; Blumenthal, J.A.; Frasure-Smith, N.; Kaufmann, P.G.; Lespérance, F.; Mark, D.B.; Sheps, D.S.; Taylor, C.B.; Froelicher, E.S. AHA science advisory. Depression and coronary heart disease. Recommendations for screening, referral, and treatment. A science advisory from the American Heart Association Prevention Committee to the Council on Cardiovascular Nursing, Council on Clinical Cardiology, Council on Epidemiology and Prevention, and Interdisciplinary Council on Quality of Care Outcomes Research. Endorsed by the American Psychiatric Association. *Prog. Cardiovasc. Nurs.* **2009**, *24*, 19–26.
18. Linden, W.; Vodermaier, A.; Mackenzie, R.; Greig, D. Anxiety and depression after cancer diagnosis: Prevalence rates by cancer type, gender, and age. *J. Affect. Disord.* **2012**, *141*, 343–351. [CrossRef]
19. Zipfel, S.; Löwe, B.; Paschke, T.; Immel, B.; Lange, R.; Zimmermann, R.; Herzog, W.; Bergmann, G. Psychological distress in patients awaiting heart transplantation. *J. Psychosom. Res.* **1998**, *45*, 465–470. [CrossRef]
20. Renoux, C.; Vahey, S.; Dell'Aniello, S.; Boivin, J.F. Association of Selective Serotonin Reuptake Inhibitors with the Risk for Spontaneous Intracranial Hemorrhage. *JAMA Neurol.* **2017**, *74*, 173–180. [CrossRef]
21. Schalekamp, T.; Klungel, O.H.; Souverein, P.C.; de Boer, A. Increased bleeding risk with concurrent use of selective serotonin reuptake inhibitors and coumarins. *Arch. Intern. Med.* **2008**, *168*, 180–185. [CrossRef]
22. Hoirisch-Clapauch, S.; Nardi, A.E. Antidepressants: Bleeding or thrombosis? *Thromb. Res.* **2019**, *181* (Suppl. S1), S23–S28. [CrossRef]
23. Spina, E.; Barbieri, M.A.; Cicala, G.; Bruno, A.; de Leon, J. Clinically relevant drug interactions between newer antidepressants and oral anticoagulants. *Expert Opin. Drug Metab. Toxicol.* **2020**, *16*, 31–44. [CrossRef] [PubMed]
24. Labos, C.; Dasgupta, K.; Nedjar, H.; Turecki, G.; Rahme, E. Risk of bleeding associated with combined use of selective serotonin reuptake inhibitors and antiplatelet therapy following acute myocardial infarction. *Can. Med. Assoc. J.* **2011**, *183*, 1835–1843. [CrossRef] [PubMed]
25. Olff, M. Stress, depression and immunity: The role of defense and coping styles. *Psychiatry Res.* **1999**, *85*, 7–15. [CrossRef]
26. Wilhelm, M.J. Long-term outcome following heart transplantation: Current perspective. *J. Thorac. Dis.* **2015**, *7*, 549–551.
27. Aziz, T.; Burgess, M.; Rahman, A.N.; Campbell, C.S.; Yonan, N. Cardiac transplantation for cardiomyopathy and ischemic heart disease: Differences in outcome up to 10 years. *J. Heart Lung Transplant.* **2001**, *20*, 525–533. [CrossRef]
28. Khush, K.K.; Cherikh, W.S.; Chambers, D.C.; Harhay, M.O.; Hayes, D., Jr.; Hsich, E.; Meiser, B.; Potena, L.; Robinson, A.; Rossano, J.W.; et al. The International Thoracic Organ Transplant Registry of the International Society for Heart and Lung Transplantation: Thirty-sixth adult heart transplantation report-2019; focus theme: Donor and recipient size match. *J. Heart Lung Transplant.* **2019**, *38*, 1056–1066. [CrossRef]

29. De Santo, L.S.; Marra, C.; De Feo, M.; Amarelli, C.; Romano, G.; Cotrufo, M. The impact of gender on heart transplantation outcomes: A single center experience. *Ital. Heart J.* **2002**, *3*, 419–423.
30. Gonzalez, M.H.; Acharya, D.; Lee, S.; Leacche, M.; Boeve, T.; Manandhar-Shrestha, N.; Jovinge, S.; Loyaga-Rendon, R.Y. Improved survival after heart transplantation in patients bridged with extracorporeal membrane oxygenation in the new allocation system. *J. Heart Lung Transplant.* **2021**, *40*, 149–157. [CrossRef]
31. Mihaljevic, T.; Jarrett, C.M.; Gonzalez-Stawinski, G.; Smedira, N.G.; Nowicki, E.R.; Thuita, L.; Mountis, M.; Blackstone, E.H. Mechanical circulatory support after heart transplantation. *Eur. J. Cardiothorac. Surg.* **2012**, *41*, 200–206. [CrossRef]

Disclaimer/Publisher's Note: The statements, opinions and data contained in all publications are solely those of the individual author(s) and contributor(s) and not of MDPI and/or the editor(s). MDPI and/or the editor(s) disclaim responsibility for any injury to people or property resulting from any ideas, methods, instructions or products referred to in the content.

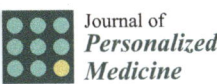

Article

Resolved Proteinuria May Attenuate the Risk of Heart Failure: A Nationwide Population-Based Cohort Study

Yoonkyung Chang [1], Min Kyoung Kang [2], Moo-Seok Park [2], Gwang-Hyun Leem [3] and Tae-Jin Song [2,*]

[1] Department of Neurology, Mokdong Hospital, Ewha Womans University College of Medicine, Seoul 08209, Republic of Korea; ykchang@ewha.ac.kr
[2] Department of Neurology, Seoul Hospital, Ewha Womans University College of Medicine, Seoul 07804, Republic of Korea; yen101@ewha.ac.kr (M.K.K.); strokesolved@ewha.ac.kr (M.-S.P.)
[3] Ewha Medical Research Institute, Ewha Womans University, Seoul 07804, Republic of Korea; shalomlkh@ewha.ac.kr
* Correspondence: knstar@ewha.ac.kr; Tel.: +82-2-6986-4478

Abstract: Although proteinuria is a risk factor for heart failure (HF), proteinuria can be reversible or persistent. Our objective was to explore the link between changes in the proteinuria status and the risk of HF. We included participants from a Korean national health screening cohort who underwent health examinations in 2003–2004 and 2005–2006 and had no history of HF. Participants were categorized into four groups: proteinuria-free, proteinuria-resolved, proteinuria-developed, and proteinuria-persistent. The outcome of interest was the occurrence of HF. The study included 1,703,651 participants, among whom 17,543 (1.03%) were in the proteinuria-resolved group and 4585 (0.27%) were in the proteinuria-persistent group. After a median follow-up period of 14.04 years (interquartile range 14.19–15.07), HF occurred in 75,064 (4.41%) participants. A multivariable Cox proportional hazards regression analysis indicated that the proteinuria-persistent group had a higher risk of HF compared with the proteinuria-free group (hazard ratio (HR): 2.19, 95% confidence interval (CI): 2.03–2.36, $p < 0.001$). In a further pairwise comparison analysis, participants in the proteinuria-resolved group had a relatively low risk of HF compared with those in the proteinuria-persistent group (HR: 0.64, 95% CI: 0.58–0.70, $p < 0.001$). In conclusion, the risk of HF can change with alterations in the proteinuria status.

Keywords: proteinuria; heart failure; dipstick test; urinalysis; epidemiology

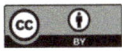

1. Introduction

Heart failure (HF) is a clinical syndrome characterized by a decline in cardiac contractility, which is often accompanied by impaired ejection of blood from the heart or compromised ventricular filling [1]. This condition is a global health concern, and its prevalence continues to surge worldwide [2]. Despite significant advancements in the development of treatment strategies, morbidity and mortality rates linked to HF remain stubbornly high [2]. Hence, there is a pressing need to comprehensively identify the various risk factors associated with HF. Established risk factors include well-documented contributors such as hypertension, diabetes mellitus, coronary artery occlusive disease, the formation of aortic atheromas, obesity, as well as the consumption of alcohol and tobacco products [3–5]. These factors play pivotal roles in the pathogenesis of HF and are crucial targets for intervention. Indeed, by adopting healthier lifestyle habits and diligently managing these cardiovascular risk factors, individuals can significantly reduce their susceptibility to developing HF. However, there remains a critical knowledge gap regarding additional modifiable factors associated with the HF risk.

The acknowledgment of elevated protein levels in the urine, referred to as proteinuria, as a risk factor for cardiovascular diseases and mortality is becoming progressively evident [6,7]. Understanding the mechanisms underlying excessive protein excretion reveals a complex interplay, including heightened glomerular filtration, insufficient tubular absorption or overflow, and augmented secretion. Notably, proteinuria stands out as a significant risk factor for stroke and coronary diseases, independently of other cardiovascular risk factors [8,9]. This multifaceted relationship between proteinuria and adverse cardiovascular outcomes underscores its critical role in the realm of cardiovascular health. Moreover, proteinuria is not limited to its association with immediate cardiovascular risks; it also serves as a harbinger of future disease states, including hypertension, diabetes, and HF [6]. Furthermore, the presence of proteinuria plays a pivotal role in determining the incidence of HF itself [7]. Intriguingly, proteinuria can manifest over time or, conversely, it can be resolved through risk correction or targeted treatment interventions. This dynamic nature of proteinuria suggests that it could indeed be a modifiable factor in the development of heart failure, offering a potential avenue for proactive intervention and prevention. Among the many tests available to measure proteinuria, dipstick testing is commonly used in screening [10]. This test can measure urinary protein exceeding 300 to 500 mg/day. If there are no other factors that can cause false-positive tests (concentrated urine, alkaline urine, hematuria, iodinated contrast agents, exercise, infection, etc.), the dipstick test should be repeated. If the second test result is negative, patients are reassured. However, transient proteinuria is also known to be a risk factor for cardiovascular and cerebrovascular diseases [11,12]. Despite this knowledge, large-scale studies examining changes in the HF risk based on alterations or the persistence of proteinuria remain conspicuously absent.

We hypothesized that the HF risk varies with a change in the proteinuria status. Our aim was to explore the correlation between shifts in the proteinuria status and the risk of heart failure within the context of a comprehensive nationwide, population-based, longitudinal study.

2. Materials and Methods

The Korean National Health Insurance System (NHIS) database includes patient-level information about demographics, socioeconomic status, diagnoses, and treatment modalities. Additionally, nationwide health examination data and healthcare institution data are available through the NHIS. NHIS subscribers are recommended to undergo standardized medical health examinations every two years. We included participants from the NHIS–National Health Screening (NHIS-HEALS) cohort. The NHIS-HEALS cohort enrolled participants who underwent medical health screening. We gathered information on their demographics, habits, including the consumption of alcohol, tobacco, regular exercise, income, weight, height, and comorbidities. This study was approved by the Institutional Review Board of the Ewha Womans University Seoul Hospital (approval number: SEUMC 2023-03-017, design of the study: 2 February 2023, IRB approval: 22 March 2023, first draft of the manuscript: 6 May 2023).

We screened all 1,878,329 individuals who had two repeated health examinations in 2003–2004 and 2005–2006, respectively. Records with absent data for variables of interest (n = 121,371) and those with HF (n = 53,307) were excluded. A total of 1,703,651 participants were included in the study (Figure 1).

Proteinuria was confirmed by dipstick urinalysis on urine samples collected in the morning after overnight fasting. Dipstick urinalysis measures proteins using Bromphenol blue indicator dye and is most sensitive to albumin. The measurement method is to put midstream urine in a container and wet a test strip. After removing any excess urine from the soaked test strip, the reading is taken approximately one minute later. The value is determined by comparing the strip's color with a numerical chart, and the results are categorized as follows: negative, 1+ (30 mg/dL), 2+ (100 mg/dL), 3+ (300 mg/dL), and 4+ (>1000 mg/dL). Participants classified the dipstick proteinuria results into two categories: "no proteinuria" and "overt proteinuria ($\geq$ 1+)." Subsequently, study participants were grouped into four categories based on the presence of proteinuria between two consecutive health examinations: (1) "proteinuria-free", (2) "proteinuria-resolved" (participants with proteinuria at the first screening but not at the second screening), (3) "proteinuria-developed" (participants with developed proteinuria at the second screening), and (4) "proteinuria-persistent".

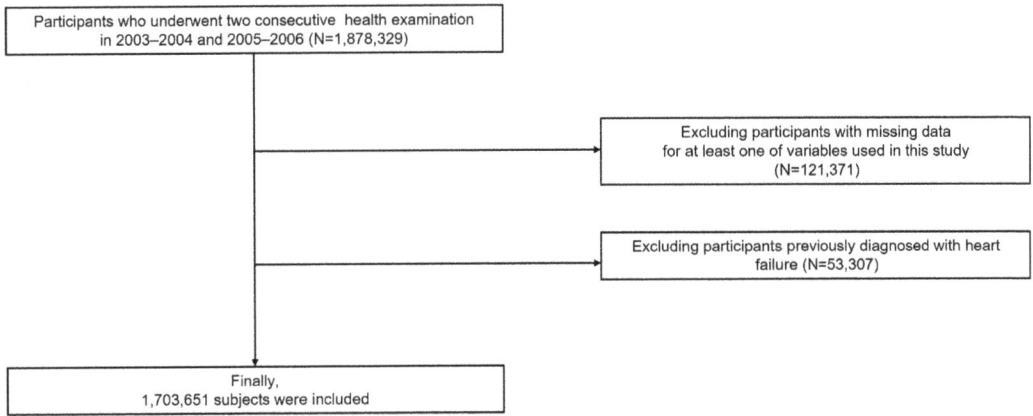

Figure 1. Flow chart of the study participants.

The index date corresponded to the health examination date. In cases where individuals underwent multiple examinations between 2005 and 2006, the most recent findings were used for the statistical analysis. The primary outcome of interest was the incidence of heart failure, defined as a participant with a minimum of two claims for HF. It is noteworthy that the diagnostic accuracy of the ICD-10 code (I50) for HF in the NHIS has been rigorously proven and employed in previous research studies [13]. Follow-up was conducted on 31 December 2020 or at the occurrence of HF or death. The study collected various covariates concerning the index date, including age, sex, body mass index (BMI), and family income. Additionally, data on alcohol consumption (frequency per week), tobacco use (none, former, or current), and regular exercise (frequency per week) were gathered through a self-reported questionnaire. Comorbidities were determined using the following criteria. Diabetes mellitus was defined as at least one claim with diagnostic codes (ICD-10 E11–14) with antidiabetic agents or two or more claims with diagnostic codes or a fasting serum glucose level ≥ 7.0 mmol/L or by self-report. Dyslipidemia was defined as at least one claim with diagnostic codes (ICD-10 E78) with related medication or two or more claims with diagnostic codes or a total cholesterol level ≥ 240 mg/dL. Cancer was defined as one or more inpatient claims with diagnostic codes (ICD-10 C00–97) or at least three outpatient claims, along with the specific registration codes 'V027' or 'V193–4'. Renal disease was defined as having two or more claims with diagnostic codes (ICD-10 N17-19, I12-13, E082, E102, E112, E132) or an estimated glomerular filtration rate of less than 60 mL/min/1.73 m^2. The Charlson Comorbidity Index was calculated as previously described [14–16]. For the covariates, findings from the most recent health examinations were applied.

Baseline characteristics were assessed utilizing the Chi-square test for categorical variables and analysis of variance, complemented by the Bonferroni post hoc analysis for continuous variables. To evaluate the association between alterations in the proteinuria status and the incidence of heart failure, Kaplan–Meier survival curves were employed, with statistical significance determined using the log-rank test. Hazard ratios (HRs) were determined using the Cox proportional hazards regression with adjustments for confounding variables. The multivariable Cox regression analysis involved adjusting for the following covariates: model 1, age and sex; model 2, variables in model 1, BMI, income, smoking, alcohol, physical activity, and comorbid diseases (diabetes mellitus, hypertension, dyslipidemia, cancer, and renal disease); model 3, variables in model 2 and the Charlson Comorbidity Index. HRs and 95% confidence intervals (CIs) were used to present the findings of the Cox regression analysis. The assumption of the proportionality of hazards was tested using

Schoenfeld residuals, and no violations were detected. A pairwise comparison analysis was used to compare the HF risk among individuals who experienced proteinuria resolution or development. A landmark analysis was performed by excluding participants with HF within one year from the index date. All statistical analyses were conducted using SAS, version 9.2 (SAS Institute, Cary, NC, USA) with the statistical significance indicated by p-values < 0.05.

3. Results

The study included 1,703,651 participants, among whom 1,661,965 (97.55%) were in the proteinuria-free group, 17,543 (1.03%) were in the proteinuria-resolved group, 19,558 (1.15%) were in the proteinuria-developed group, and 4585 (0.27%) were in the proteinuria-persistent group. The respective second health screenings were performed after a median of 21.5 months (interquartile range, 11.1–25.5 months). The mean age was 43.94 ± 12.05 years, and 69.14% of participants were men. Compared with the proteinuria-free group, the proteinuria-persistent group consisted of older men with higher BMIs and a higher likelihood of comorbidities (Table 1).

Table 1. Baseline characteristics of the study population according to the proteinuria status.

Variable	Total	Proteinuria-Free (−/−)	Proteinuria-Resolved (+/−)	Proteinuria-Developed (−/+)	Proteinuria-Persistent (+/+)	p-Value
Number of participants (%)	1,703,651	1,661,965 (97.55)	17,543 (1.03)	19,558 (1.15)	4585 (0.27)	
Age, years	43.94 ± 12.05	43.86 ± 12.01	46.74 ± 13.11	46.73 ± 12.99	49.26 ± 12.6	<0.001
Sex						<0.001
Men	1,177,934 (69.14)	1,150,367 (69.22)	11,031 (62.88)	12,928 (66.10)	3608 (78.69)	
Women	525,717 (30.86)	511,598 (30.78)	6512 (37.12)	6630 (33.90)	977 (21.31)	
Body mass index (kg/m^2)	23.62 ± 3.03	23.61 ± 3.02	24.13 ± 3.32	24.17 ± 3.44	24.94 ± 3.37	<0.001
Household income						<0.001
Q1, lowest	254,366 (14.93)	247,563 (14.90)	3038 (17.32)	3135 (16.03)	630 (13.74)	
Q2	632,196 (37.11)	617,708 (37.17)	6240 (35.57)	6872 (35.14)	1376 (30.01)	
Q3	562,916 (33.04)	549,527 (33.06)	5498 (31.34)	6282 (32.12)	1609 (35.09)	
Q4, highest	254,173 (14.92)	247,167 (14.87)	2767 (15.77)	3269 (16.71)	970 (21.16)	
Smoking						<0.001
Never	980,235 (57.54)	954,998 (57.46)	10,904 (62.16)	11,807 (60.37)	2526 (55.09)	
Former	212,652 (12.48)	207,536 (12.49)	2071 (11.81)	2356 (12.05)	689 (15.03)	
Current	510,764 (29.98)	499,431 (30.05)	4568 (26.04)	5395 (27.58)	1370 (29.88)	
Alcohol consumption (days/week)						<0.001
<3	1,139,835 (66.91)	1,111,388 (66.87)	12,133 (69.16)	13,292 (67.96)	3022 (65.91)	
≥3	563,816 (33.09)	550,577 (33.13)	5410 (30.84)	6266 (32.04)	1563 (34.09)	
Regular exercise (days/week)						<0.001
<3	1,374,142 (80.66)	1341,444 (80.71)	13,597 (77.51)	15,552 (79.52)	3549 (77.40)	
≥3	329,509 (19.34)	320,521 (19.29)	3946 (22.49)	4006 (20.48)	1036 (22.60)	
Comorbidities (%)						
Hypertension	769,339 (45.16)	744,298 (44.78)	10,067 (57.38)	11,373 (58.15)	3601 (78.54)	<0.001
Diabetes mellitus	239,866 (14.08)	228,364 (13.74)	4482 (25.55)	5188 (26.53)	1832 (39.96)	<0.001
Dyslipidemia	421,156 (24.72)	405,688 (24.41)	6250 (35.63)	6871 (35.13)	2347 (51.19)	<0.001
Atrial fibrillation	4448 (0.26)	4234 (0.25)	76 (0.43)	104 (0.53)	34 (0.74)	<0.001
Cancer	31,454 (1.85)	30,290 (1.82)	493 (2.81)	504 (2.58)	167 (3.64)	<0.001
Renal disease	16,806 (0.99)	14,682 (0.88)	785 (4.47)	699 (3.57)	640 (13.96)	<0.001
Charlson Comorbidity Index						<0.001
0	677,492 (39.77)	664,172 (39.96)	5674 (32.34)	6459 (33.02)	1187 (25.89)	
1	691,773 (40.61)	676,615 (40.71)	6467 (36.86)	7314 (37.4)	1377 (30.03)	
≥2	334,386 (19.63)	321,178 (19.33)	5402 (30.79)	5785 (29.58)	2021 (44.08)	
Follow-up duration (years)	14.04 ± 2.36	14.06 ± 2.33	13.56 ± 3.08	13.38 ± 3.33	12.6 ± 3.90	<0.001

Data are presented as the mean ± standard deviation or number (percentage). Q, Quartile.

The baseline characteristics of the participants according to the heart failure are summarized in Supplementary Table S1. The heart failure group was older, obese, had more frequent consumption of alcohol, and had multiple comorbidities.

After a median follow-up period of 14.04 ± 2.36 years, HF occurred in 75,064 (4.41%) participants. Among the proteinuria groups, HF occurred most frequently in the proteinuria-persistent group (Figure 2). The Kaplan–Meier curve showed that there were no significant differences between the proteinuria-resolved group and the proteinuria-developed group. The multivariate analysis indicated that participants in the proteinuria-persistent group had a higher risk of HF than participants in the proteinuria-free group (HR: 2.19, 95% CI: 2.03–2.36, $p < 0.001$, Table 2, model 3) after adjusting for age, sex, and comorbid diseases. Participants in the proteinuria-resolved (HR: 1.31, 95% CI: 1.24–1.38, $p < 0.001$) and proteinuria-developed (HR: 1.52, 95% CI: 1.44–1.59, $p < 0.001$) groups also had a higher risk of HF than those in the proteinuria-free group. In a further pairwise comparison, participants in the proteinuria-resolved group had a lower risk of HF than participants in the proteinuria-persistent group (HR: 0.64, 95% CI: 0.58–0.70, $p < 0.001$). The risk of HF in the proteinuria-developed was higher than that in the proteinuria-free group (HR: 1.52, 95% CI: 1.45–1.60, $p < 0.001$) according to the multivariable analysis (Table 3, model 3). Additionally, when the risk of HF was analyzed according to the degree of proteinuria, the risk of HF was higher in the 4+ proteinuria group than in the proteinuria-negative group (Supplementary Table S2). The risk of HF increased as the degree of proteinuria increased, and this trend was the same in the first (2003–2004) and second (2004–2005) health examinations.

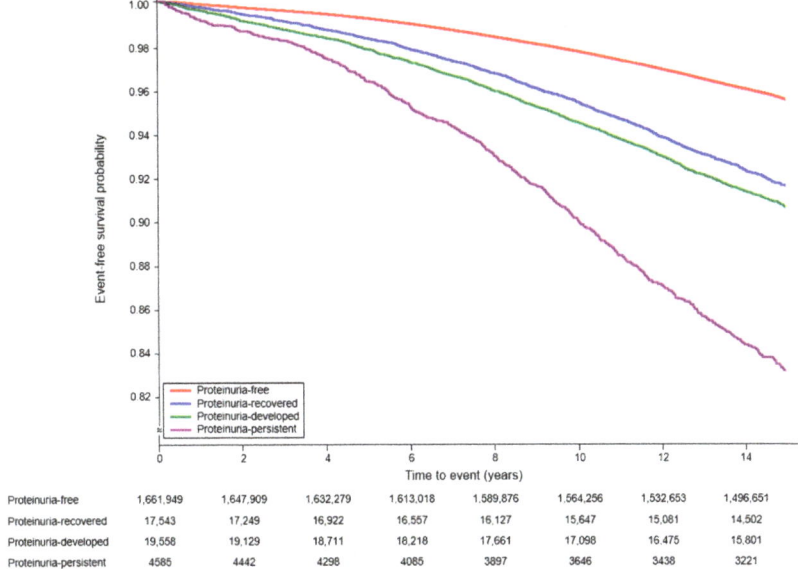

Figure 2. Kaplan–Meier survival curves associated with the proteinuria status and risk of heart failure occurrence.

Table 2. Multivariable Cox analysis for the incidence of heart failure according to changes in the proteinuria status.

Proteinuria Status	Total (N)	Heart Failure (N)	IR (per 1000)	HR (95% Confidence Interval)		
				Model 1	Model 2	Model 3
Free	1,661,965	71,276	3.05	1 (ref)	1 (ref)	1 (ref)
Resolved	17,543	1386	5.83	1.93 (1.83, 2.03)	1.32 (1.25, 1.39)	1.31 (1.24, 1.38)
Developed	19,558	1708	6.53	2.16 (2.06, 2.27)	1.53 (1.46, 1.60)	1.52 (1.44, 1.59)
Persistent	4585	694	12.02	4.06 (3.77, 4.38)	2.23 (2.06, 2.40)	2.19 (2.03, 2.36)
		p-value		<0.001	<0.001	<0.001

Model 1, age and sex. Model 2, variables in model 1, body mass index, income, smoking, alcohol, exercise, history of diabetes mellitus, dyslipidemia, atrial fibrillation, cancer, and renal disease. Model 3, variables in model 2 and the Charlson Comorbidity Index. IR, incidence rate; HR, hazard ratio; CI, confidence interval.

Table 3. Pairwise comparison for the incidence of heart failure according to changes in the proteinuria status.

	Model 1			Model 2			Model 3		
	HR	95% CI	p-value	HR	95% CI	p-value	HR	95% CI	p-value
Resolved vs. Free (ref)	1.93	(1.83, 2.03)	<0.001	1.32	(1.26, 1.40)	<0.001	1.31	(1.24, 1.38)	<0.001
Developed vs. Free (ref)	2.17	(2.07, 2.27)	<0.001	1.53	(1.46, 1.60)	<0.001	1.52	(1.45, 1.59)	<0.001
Resolved vs. Persistent (ref)	0.48	(0.44, 0.52)	<0.001	0.64	(0.58, 0.70)	<0.001	0.64	(0.58, 0.70)	<0.001
Developed vs. Persistent (ref)	0.54	(0.49, 0.59)	<0.001	0.73	(0.67, 0.80)	<0.001	0.74	(0.68, 0.81)	<0.001

Model 1, age and sex. Model 2, variables in model 1, body mass index, income, smoking, alcohol, exercise, history of diabetes mellitus, dyslipidemia, atrial fibrillation, cancer, and renal disease. Model 3, variables in model 2 and the Charlson Comorbidity Index; vs., versus; HR, hazard ratio; CI, confidence interval.

A subgroup analysis performed in regard to the presence of renal disease showed that the risk of HF was higher in the proteinuria-persistent group among participants with and without renal disease (with renal disease, HR: 2.61, 95% CI: 2.22–3.08, $p < 0.001$; without renal disease, HR: 2.05, 95% CI: 1.88–2.23, $p < 0.001$, Supplementary Table S3, Supplementary Figure S1). The proteinuria-resolved (with renal disease, HR: 1.64, 95% CI: 1.39–1.93, $p < 0.001$; without renal disease, HR: 1.27, 95% CI: 1.20–1.35, $p < 0.001$), and proteinuria-developed (with renal disease, HR: 1.47, 95% CI: 1.4–1.55, $p < 0.001$; without renal disease, HR: 2.05, 95% CI: 1.88–2.23, $p < 0.001$) groups also had a higher risk of HF, regardless of the presence of renal disease. The landmark analysis indicated a consistent association between the proteinuria status and the risk of HF (HR: 2.19, 95% CI: 2.03–2.36, $p < 0.001$ in model 3, Supplementary Table S4). The proteinuria-resolved (HR: 1.30, 95% CI: 1.24–1.38, $p < 0.001$ in model 3) and proteinuria-developed groups (HR: 1.51, 95% CI: 1.43–1.58, $p < 0.001$ in model 3) showed an elevated risk of HF compared to the proteinuria-free group.

4. Discussion

Our study's key findings indicate that the HF risk depends on changes in the proteinuria status. The risk of heart failure was notably elevated in cases where proteinuria was newly identified or persistent. Interestingly, we also observed that the risk of heart failure decreased when proteinuria had been resolved.

The presence and severity of proteinuria are strong predictors of the future HF risk, regardless of the estimated glomerular filtration rate or other traditional cardiovascular risk factors [17–19]. The Heart Outcomes Prevention Evaluation study was a cohort study with individuals aged 55 or older with cardiovascular disease or its risk factors. After a median 4.5-year follow-up period, microalbuminuria was associated with an increased risk of major cardiovascular events, heart failure, and mortality in patients with and without diabetes mellitus [18]. In a large number ($n = 10,975$) of prospective observational studies of HF-free participants (Atherosclerosis Risk in Communities (ARIC) Study), albuminuria was associated with a future risk of HF [19]. This study categorized the urinary albumin/creatinine ratio as optimal, intermediate normal, high normal, microalbuminuria, and macroalbuminuria. The results showed that the intermediate normal and high normal groups had higher risks of HF compared to the optimal group (adjusted HR, 1.54; 95% CI, 1.12–2.11, adjusted HR, 1.91; 95% CI, 1.38–2.66, respectively). Furthermore, a Japanese atrial fibrillation registry study found proteinuria to be significantly associated with an increased risk of HF among patients with atrial fibrillation [20]. These complementary findings from diverse cohorts emphasize the robustness of the relationship between proteinuria and heart failure, transcending geographical and clinical boundaries. Notably, the presence of proteinuria has consistently emerged as a red flag, signaling an increased susceptibility to various cardiovascular risk factors and the associated mortality risks linked to these factors. Among these risk factors are hypertension, diabetes mellitus, and ischemic heart disease [6]. However, it is imperative to recognize the dynamic nature of the parameters within these cohorts. Our study contributes a fresh perspective to this discourse by revealing a novel finding: the risk of heart failure escalates significantly when proteinuria persists for a duration of at least 2 years. This temporal dimension adds an important layer of insight into the evolving nature of heart failure risk and the potential impact of sustained proteinuria.

In our study, a noteworthy observation emerged: as proteinuria improved, the risk of heart failure (HF) also demonstrated a significant decrease. This finding underscores the potential modifiability of this risk factor, offering a promising avenue for preventive strategies against HF. While there exists a well-established cadre of modifiable risk factors associated with HF, encompassing hypertension, diabetes mellitus, obesity, smoking, and dyslipidemia [21], it is crucial to incorporate proteinuria into the framework of a comprehensive prevention and management strategy for HF. Despite the widely acknowledged significance of proteinuria as a risk factor for HF, relatively few studies have delved into the question of whether the risk of HF diminishes with the improvement of proteinuria. Our research fills this knowledge gap by shedding light on this critical aspect. Intriguingly, our findings revealed that both the group with resolved proteinuria and the group that developed proteinuria had similar risks for HF occurrence. This intriguing revelation underscores the idea that transient proteinuria, which ultimately resolves, may pose a lower risk of HF compared to persistent proteinuria. This shift in risk may, in part, be attributed to the duration of proteinuria (new versus persistent), suggesting that the timeline of proteinuria can influence the risk of HF development. Considering these findings, the potential of correcting proteinuria to reduce the risk of future HF takes on paramount significance.

Although we may not be able to provide an exact mechanism for the association between persistent or improved proteinuria and changes in HF risk, we can propose the following hypotheses. The presence of proteinuria can lead to structural changes in the heart, such as left ventricular hypertrophy [22]. Left ventricular hypertrophy is characterized by the thickening of the walls of the heart's primary pumping chamber, a response that can occur due to heightened pressure and volume stresses. Left ventricular hypertrophy is associated with an increased risk of HF development. A thickened and stiffened left ventricle may lead to impaired relaxation and filling of the heart, resulting in diastolic dysfunction, which is a common form of HF [23]. Moreover, attenuated proteinuria may reflect improved kidney function and a reduction in the underlying inflammatory processes that contribute to HF development. Additionally, proteinuria-associated conditions, such as hypertension and diabetes, can also increase the risk of HF through various mechanisms, such as the promotion of inflammation, endothelial dysfunction, and oxidative stress [24]. Overall, the association between proteinuria and an increased risk of HF is likely multifactorial, involving both structural changes in the heart and the presence of comorbidities that promote HF development.

Our study had several limitations. Although this was a longitudinal study, it is not possible to confirm a causal relationship with a retrospective cohort study. Since our dataset only included Asian participants, generalization to other ethnicities is difficult. We confirmed proteinuria using a validated dipstick test, but we could not suggest a direct cause of proteinuria. Additionally, the presence of proteinuria was tested by a urine dipstick test instead of through 24 h urine collection. In a former study of the diagnostic accuracy of the urine dipstick test (1+ or higher), the sensitivity was 57.8% and the specificity was 95.4% [25]. A further study using 24 h urine collection is needed to provide stronger evidence of proteinuria improvement and the risk of HF.

5. Conclusions

The risk of HF can change with changes in the proteinuria status. Proteinuria can be considered a modifiable risk factor for HF.

Supplementary Materials: The following are available online at https://www.mdpi.com/article/10.3390/jpm13121662/s1, Table S1: Baseline characteristics of the study participants according to the heart failure incidence, Table S2: Multivariable Cox analysis for the incidence of heart failure according to the proteinuria significance, Table S3: Multivariable Cox analysis for the incidence of heart failure according to the proteinuria status, Table S4: Multivariable Cox analysis for the incidence of heart failure according to changes in the proteinuria status (landmark analysis), Figure S1: Subgroup analysis for the association between the proteinuria status and heart failure occurrence.

Author Contributions: Conceptualization, T.-J.S.; methodology, G.-H.L. and T.-J.S.; software, G.-H.L. and T.-J.S.; validation, Y.C., G.-H.L. and T.-J.S.; formal analysis, G.-H.L. and T.-J.S.; investigation, Y.C. and T.-J.S.; resources, T.-J.S.; data curation, G.-H.L.; writing—original draft preparation, Y.C. and T.-J.S.; writing—review and editing, Y.C., M.K.K., M.-S.P., G.-H.L. and T.-J.S.; visualization, Y.C.; supervision, T.-J.S.; project administration, T.-J.S.; funding acquisition, Y.C. and T.-J.S. All authors have read and agreed to the published version of the manuscript.

Funding: This project was supported by a grant from the Basic Science Research Program through the National Research Foundation of Korea funded by the Ministry of Education (2021R1I1A1A01059868 to YC). This work was supported by the Institute of Information & Communications Technology Planning & Evaluation (IITP) grant funded by the Korean government (MSIT) (2022-0-00621 to TJS, Development of artificial intelligence technology that provides dialog-based multi-modal explainability). This research was supported by a grant from the Korea Health Technology R&D Project through the Korea Health Industry Development Institute (KHIDI), funded by the Ministry of Health & Welfare, Republic of Korea (grant number: HI22C073600, RS-2023-00262087 to TJS).

Institutional Review Board Statement: The study was conducted according to the guidelines of the Declaration of Helsinki and approved by the Institutional Review Board of Ewha Womans University College of Medicine (SEUMC-2023-03-017).

Informed Consent Statement: Patient consent was waived due to the fully anonymized dataset.

Data Availability Statement: The data that support the findings of this study are available from NHIS-HEALS, but restrictions apply to the availability of these data, which were used under license for the study reported herein and, hence, are not publicly available. Data are, however, available from the authors upon reasonable request and with permission from the National Health Insurance System.

Conflicts of Interest: The authors declare no conflict of interest. The funders had no role in the design of the study; in the collection, analyses, or interpretation of data; in the writing of the manuscript, or in the decision to publish the results.

References

1. Tan, L.B.; Williams, S.G.; Tan, D.K.; Cohen-Solal, A. So many definitions of heart failure: Are they all universally valid? A critical appraisal. *Expert Rev. Cardiovasc. Ther.* **2010**, *8*, 217–228. [CrossRef] [PubMed]
2. Savarese, G.; Lund, L.H. Global Public Health Burden of Heart Failure. *Card. Fail. Rev.* **2017**, *3*, 7–11. [CrossRef] [PubMed]
3. Djoussé, L.; Driver, J.A.; Gaziano, J.M. Relation between modifiable lifestyle factors and lifetime risk of heart failure. *JAMA* **2009**, *302*, 394–400. [CrossRef] [PubMed]
4. Bui, A.L.; Horwich, T.B.; Fonarow, G.C. Epidemiology and risk profile of heart failure. *Nat. Rev. Cardiol.* **2011**, *8*, 30–41. [CrossRef] [PubMed]
5. Inamdar, A.A.; Inamdar, A.C. Heart Failure: Diagnosis, Management and Utilization. *J. Clin. Med.* **2016**, *5*, 62. [CrossRef]
6. Currie, G.; Delles, C. Proteinuria and its relation to cardiovascular disease. *Int. J. Nephrol. Renovasc. Dis.* **2013**, *7*, 13–24. [CrossRef]
7. Liang, W.; Liu, Q.; Wang, Q.Y.; Yu, H.; Yu, J. Albuminuria and Dipstick Proteinuria for Predicting Mortality in Heart Failure: A Systematic Review and Meta-Analysis. *Front. Cardiovasc. Med.* **2021**, *8*, 665831. [CrossRef]

8. Kumai, Y.; Kamouchi, M.; Hata, J.; Ago, T.; Kitayama, J.; Nakane, H.; Sugimori, H.; Kitazono, T. Proteinuria and clinical outcomes after ischemic stroke. *Neurology* **2012**, *78*, 1909–1915. [CrossRef]
9. Kelly, D.M.; Rothwell, P.M. Proteinuria as an independent predictor of stroke: Systematic review and meta-analysis. *Int. J. Stroke* **2020**, *15*, 29–38. [CrossRef]
10. Wen, C.P.; Yang, Y.C.; Tsai, M.K.; Wen, S.F. Urine dipstick to detect trace proteinuria: An underused tool for an underappreciated risk marker. *Am. J. Kidney Dis.* **2011**, *58*, 1–3. [CrossRef]
11. Wang, A.; Jiang, R.; Su, Z.; Zhang, J.; Zhao, X.; Wu, S.; Guo, X. Association of Persistent, Incident, and Remittent Proteinuria With Stroke Risk in Patients With Diabetes Mellitus or Prediabetes Mellitus. *J. Am. Heart Assoc.* **2017**, *6*, e006178. [CrossRef] [PubMed]
12. Madison, J.R.; Spies, C.; Schatz, I.J.; Masaki, K.; Chen, R.; Yano, K.; Curb, J.D. Proteinuria and risk for stroke and coronary heart disease during 27 years of follow-up: The Honolulu Heart Program. *Arch. Intern. Med.* **2006**, *166*, 884–889. [CrossRef] [PubMed]
13. Choi, E.-K. Cardiovascular Research Using the Korean National Health Information Database. *Korean Circ. J.* **2020**, *50*, 754–772. [CrossRef]
14. Charlson, M.E.; Carrozzino, D.; Guidi, J.; Patierno, C. Charlson Comorbidity Index: A Critical Review of Clinimetric Properties. *Psychother. Psychosom.* **2022**, *91*, 8–35. [CrossRef] [PubMed]
15. Hwang, J.; Yi, H.; Jang, M.; Kim, J.G.; Kwon, S.U.; Kim, N.; Lee, E.J. Air Pollution and Subarachnoid Hemorrhage Mortality: A Stronger Association in Women than in Men. *J. Stroke* **2022**, *24*, 429–432. [CrossRef]
16. Jung, S.; Jung, G.; Kim, D.; Oh, J.; Choi, K. Epidemiology of Chronic Inflammatory Demyelinating Polyneuropathy in South Korea: A Population-Based Study. *J. Clin. Neurol.* **2023**, *19*, 558–564. [CrossRef]
17. Khan, M.S.; Shahid, I.; Anker, S.D.; Fonarow, G.C.; Fudim, M.; Hall, M.E.; Hernandez, A.; Morris, A.A.; Shafi, T.; Weir, M.R.; et al. Albuminuria and Heart Failure: JACC State-of-the-Art Review. *J. Am. Coll. Cardiol.* **2023**, *81*, 270–282. [CrossRef]
18. Gerstein, H.C.; Mann, J.F.; Yi, Q.; Zinman, B.; Dinneen, S.F.; Hoogwerf, B.; Hallé, J.P.; Young, J.; Rashkow, A.; Joyce, C.; et al. Albuminuria and risk of cardiovascular events, death, and heart failure in diabetic and nondiabetic individuals. *JAMA* **2001**, *286*, 421–426. [CrossRef]
19. Blecker, S.; Matsushita, K.; Köttgen, A.; Loehr, L.R.; Bertoni, A.G.; Boulware, L.E.; Coresh, J. High-normal albuminuria and risk of heart failure in the community. *Am. J. Kidney Dis.* **2011**, *58*, 47–55. [CrossRef]
20. Ikeda, S.; An, Y.; Iguchi, M.; Ogawa, H.; Nakanishi, Y.; Minami, K.; Ishigami, K.; Aono, Y.; Doi, K.; Hamatani, Y.; et al. Proteinuria is independently associated with heart failure events in patients with atrial fibrillation: The Fushimi AF registry. *Eur. Heart J. Qual. Care Clin. Outcomes*, **2023**; online ahead of print. [CrossRef]
21. Hamo, C.E.; Kwak, L.; Wang, D.; Florido, R.; Echouffo-Tcheugui, J.B.; Blumenthal, R.S.; Loehr, L.; Matsushita, K.; Nambi, V.; Ballantyne, C.M.; et al. Heart Failure Risk Associated With Severity of Modifiable Heart Failure Risk Factors: The ARIC Study. *J. Am. Heart Assoc.* **2022**, *11*, e021583. [CrossRef]
22. Wu, N.; Zhao, W.; Ye, K.; Li, Y.; He, M.; Lu, B.; Hu, R. Albuminuria Is Associated with Left Ventricular Hypertrophy in Patients with Early Diabetic Kidney Disease. *Int. J. Endocrinol.* **2014**, *2014*, 351945. [CrossRef] [PubMed]
23. Lorell, B.H.; Carabello, B.A. Left Ventricular Hypertrophy. *Circulation* **2000**, *102*, 470–479. [CrossRef] [PubMed]
24. Farré, A.L.; Casado, S. Heart Failure, Redox Alterations, and Endothelial Dysfunction. *Hypertension* **2001**, *38*, 1400–1405. [CrossRef] [PubMed]
25. White, S.L.; Yu, R.; Craig, J.C.; Polkinghorne, K.R.; Atkins, R.C.; Chadban, S.J. Diagnostic accuracy of urine dipsticks for detection of albuminuria in the general community. *Am. J. Kidney Dis.* **2011**, *58*, 19–28. [CrossRef]

Disclaimer/Publisher's Note: The statements, opinions and data contained in all publications are solely those of the individual author(s) and contributor(s) and not of MDPI and/or the editor(s). MDPI and/or the editor(s) disclaim responsibility for any injury to people or property resulting from any ideas, methods, instructions or products referred to in the content.

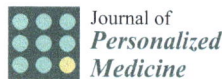

Brief Report

A Comparative Study to Investigate the Effects of Bisoprolol in Patients with Chronic Heart Failure and Hypertension When Switched from Tablets to Transdermal Patches

Akira Sezai *, Hisakuni Sekino, Makoto Taoka, Shunji Osaka and Masashi Tanaka

Department of Cardiovascular Surgery, Nihon University School of Medicine, Sekino Hospital, 30-1 Oyaguchi-kamimachi, Itabashi-ku, Tokyo 173-8610, Japan; sekinoh@sekino-hospital.com (H.S.); taoka.makoto@nihon-u.ac.jp (M.T.); osaka.shunji@nihon-u.ac.jp (S.O.)
* Correspondence: asezai.med@gmail.com; Tel.: +81-3-3972-8111; Fax: +81-3-3955-9818

Abstract: Background: Oral beta-blockers are effective for heart failure and hypertension. Here, we conducted a prospective study to investigate the efficacy of the beta-blocker bisoprolol in patients switching from the oral tablet to the transdermal patch. Methods: We studied 50 outpatients receiving oral bisoprolol for chronic heart failure and hypertension. After patients switched treatments, we measured heart rate (HR) over 24 h by Holter echocardiography as the primary endpoint. Secondary endpoints were (1) HR at 00:00, 06:00, 12:00, and 18:00, (2) the total number of premature atrial contractions (PACs) over 24 h and the incidence rate per time segment, and the total number of premature ventricular contractions (PVCs) over 24 h and the incidence rate per time segment, (3) blood pressure, (4) atrial natriuretic peptide and B-type natriuretic peptide, and (5) echocardiography. Results: Minimum, maximum, mean, and total HR over 24 h was not significantly different between the two groups. Mean and maximum HR at 06:00, total PACs, total PVCs, and PVCs at 00:00 to 05:59 and 06:00 to 11:59 were significantly lower in the patch group. Conclusion: Compared with oral bisoprolol, the bisoprolol transdermal patch lowers HR at 06:00 and inhibits the onset of PVCs during sleep and in the morning.

Keywords: bisoprolol; beta-blocker; percutaneous; transdermal patch; heart failure

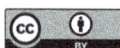

1. Introduction

The efficacy of oral beta-blockers in heart failure has been demonstrated in numerous large-scale trials, and they are one of the drugs needed for the treatment of heart failure [1,2]. Among beta-blockers, bisoprolol is preferred because it has the highest selectivity for the β_1 receptor and fewer adverse reactions in patients with bronchial asthma and diabetes [3]. Transdermally administered beta-blockers containing bisoprolol were originally developed in Japan; bisoprolol was approved for the treatment of essential hypertension in 2013, and then its indications were expanded to include tachycardiac atrial fibrillation in 2019. This drug is administered once daily to achieve a stable plasma concentration. It reportedly achieves stable blood pressure lowering and heart rate lowering effects over 24 h [4]. Moreover, Matsuoka et al. reported that the 8 mg transdermal patch maintains a sustained plasma concentration of bisoprolol while lowering the peak plasma bisoprolol concentration and has a higher trough concentration than the oral 5 mg tablet; the area under the curve of plasma concentrations was similar to that of the 5 mg oral tablet [5]. Therefore, we conducted a prospective clinical study to evaluate the effects of switching patients from oral bisoprolol tablets to bisoprolol transdermal patches by measuring pulse rates and other parameters.

2. Methods

2.1. Study Protocol

This was an open-label, non-randomized trial that lasted 6 months. Study participants were outpatients who were receiving standard treatment for chronic heart failure and hypertension, had been treated with a beta-blocker for at least 6 months, and had stable disease without dose modifications. Afterward, they switched to using a bisoprolol transdermal patch (Bisono® Tape, TOA EIYO Ltd. Astellas Pharma Inc., Tokyo, Japan). Chronic heart failure was defined as heart failure in patients currently on oral medications for the treatment of heart failure, such as diuretics, β-blockers, and renin–angiotensin system inhibitors. The data at the time of oral bisoprolol administration was used as the tablet group, and the data after switching from oral bisoprolol to the transdermal patch was used as the patch group.

Baseline data were obtained before switching from oral bisoprolol to the patch, and monitoring was continued for 6 months after the medication switch (Figure 1). Oral bisoprolol tablets were taken orally after breakfast, and a bisoprolol transdermal patch was attached to the chest or upper arm after breakfast. The comparative test doses of the bisoprolol transdermal patch and oral bisoprolol were 2 mg to 1.25 mg, 4 mg to 2.5 mg, and 8 mg to 5 mg, respectively. A Holter electrocardiogram (ECG) and echocardiography were conducted before patients switched to the bisoprolol transdermal patch at 0 months and again at 6 months.

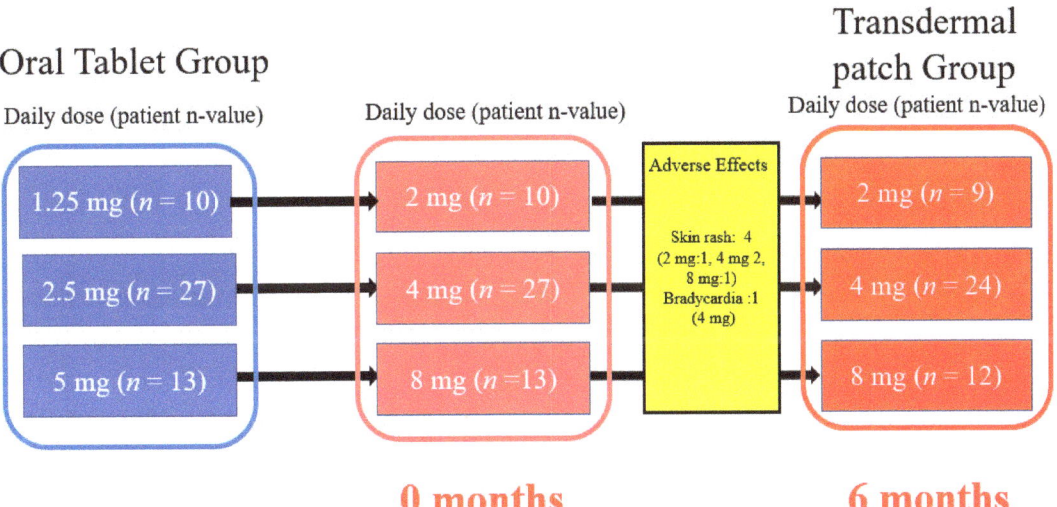

Figure 1. Study flowchart.

This study was conducted at Sekino Hospital, a logistical support hospital of the Nihon University Itabashi Hospital, according to the Declaration of Helsinki. The study details were explained to patients, and written informed consent was obtained. The study was approved by our institutional review board and registered with our Hospital Medical Information Network (study ID: UMIN000031538).

The primary endpoints were measurements of minimum, mean, maximum, and total heart rate over 24 h determined by using a Holter ECG before (at 0 months) and 6 months after the medication switch.

The secondary endpoints were as follows: (1) minimum, maximum, and mean heart rate at 00:00, 06:00, 12:00, and 18:00 measured by Holter ECG (measurements at 6:00 and 00:00 were conducted during sleep); (2) the total number of premature atrial contractions (PACs) over 24 h (excluding atrial fibrillation), the number of events in each time interval, and the total number of premature ventricular contractions (PVCs) over 24 h; (3) home blood pressure measurements (systolic and diastolic) in the early morning; (4) atrial natriuretic peptide (ANP) and B-type natriuretic peptide (BNP) levels measured at 0, 3, and 6 months; (5) echocardiography (0 months and 6 months after medication switch), left ventricular ejection (EF), fractional shortening (% FS), left ventricular end-diastolic dimension (LVDd), left ventricular end-systolic dimensions (LVDs), and the left ventricular mass index (LVMI).

The following adverse effects were recorded: hypotension, bradycardia, renal dysfunction (defined as an increase in serum Cr levels by $\geq 50\%$), hepatic dysfunction (defined as an increase in AST/ALT by $\geq 50\%$), skin reactions, and allergic reactions. The management of adverse reactions, which included the discontinuation of the bisoprolol transdermal patch, was decided by the attending physician.

2.2. Statistical Analysis

Observed values were expressed as medians and 25th and 75th percentiles. ANP and BNP were analyzed by Friedman's test, and the other variables by the Wilcoxon signed rank test. A p-value of less than 0.05 was considered statistically significant.

3. Results

Fifty patients were enrolled in this trial, and their baseline characteristics are shown in Table 1. In accordance with the study protocol, patients switched from the oral tablet to the transdermal patch and remained on it for 6 months. Five patients discontinued the transdermal patch during the study; the reasons for discontinuation were the development of skin rashes in four patients (8%) and the development of bradycardia in one patient (2%). Except for the five discontinued cases, all data were analyzed.

Table 1. Patient characteristics.

Total number of patients	50
Age (years)	75.1 ± 9.5
Sex: male, female	28, 22
Basic disease	n (%)
Ischemic heart disease	13 (26%)
Valvular disease	22 (44%)
Hypertensive heart disease	13 (26%)
Other	2 (4%)
Classification of heart failure	n (%)
HFrEF	6 (12%)
HFmrEF	5 (10%)
HFpEF	33 (66%)
HFpEF improved	6 (12%)
Risk factors	n (%)
Type 2 diabetes	18 (36%)
Dyslipidemia	41 (82%)
Hyperuricemia	25 (50%)
Atrial fibrillation	17 (34%)
Obesity	9 (18%)
Medications	n (%)
Oral bisoprolol	
1.25 mg	10 (20%)

Table 1. Cont.

2.5 mg	27 (54%)
5.0 mg	13 (26%)
Calcium antagonist	17 (34%)
Angiotensin II receptor blocker	18 (36%)
ACE inhibitor	4 (8%)
Aldosterone blocker	22 (44%)
α-blocker	5 (10%)
Diuretics	17 (34%)
Oral hypoglycemic agent	18 (36%)
Statin	42 (84%)
Ezetimibe	12 (24%)
Xanthanide oxidase antagonist	25 (50%)
Antiarrhythmic drugs	n (%)
Bepridil	4 (8%)
Disopyramide	1 (2%)
Mexiletine	10 (20%)
Pilsicanide	4 (8%)
Verapamil	2 (4%)

ACE, angiotensin-converting enzyme; HFmrEF, heart failure with mid-range ejection fraction; HFpEFm, heart failure with preserved ejection fraction; HFrEF, heart failure with reduced ejection fraction.

Primary endpoints are shown in Table 2. There were no significant differences between the two groups in the minimum, maximum, mean, and total HR over 24 h.

Table 2. Blood pressure, heart rate, premature ventricular contractions, and premature atrial contractions over 24 h before and after switching from oral bisoprolol tablets to the bisoprolol transdermal patch.

	Tablet	Patch	p Value
Systolic blood pressure (mm Hg)	127 (117, 137.5)	127.5 (116.5, 141.3)	0.674
Diastolic blood pressure (mm Hg)	71.5 (65.8, 81.3)	73.5 (66, 81)	0.977
Heart rate			
Minimum (bpm)	56 (51, 60.5)	54 (51, 61)	0.63
Mean (bpm)	73 (68.5, 80.5)	72 (66.5, 77)	0.227
Maximum (bpm)	115 (102.5, 126)	112 (97.5, 126)	0.359
Total (n)	100,865 (90,907, 109,855)	96,953 (90,365, 106,020)	0.467
PVC time segment (h)			
0–5	8 (1, 87)	4 (0, 24.5)	0.005
6–11	13 (3, 110)	8 (5, 32.5)	0.009
12–17	10 (3, 85)	13 (1, 58.5)	0.359
18–24	15 (2, 101)	15 (1, 42.5)	0.085
PAC time segment (h)			
0–5	10 (0, 46.5)	5 (0, 23.5)	0.07
6–11	8 (0, 56)	12 (0, 26)	0.062
12–17	13 (0, 53)	10 (0, 23.5)	0.269
18–24	11 (0, 28)	10 (0, 28.5)	0.33

PACs, premature atrial contractions; PVCs, premature ventricular contractions.

The results of the secondary endpoints are summarized below:

(1) The hourly heart rates are shown in Table 3. For heart rates measured at 6:00, there were no differences in the minimum heart rates between the groups ($p = 0.334$). However, the mean heart rates at 06:00 were 72.9 ± 2.1 bpm and 67.7 ± 1.6 bpm in the tablet and patch groups, respectively ($p = 0.018$), and the maximum heart rates at 06:00 were 90.0 ± 2.9 bpm and 80.6 ± 2.6 in the tablet and patch groups, respectively ($p = 0.002$). Thus, the hourly heart rate was significantly lower in the patch group than in the tablet group. No group differences were observed at other time points.

Table 3. Minimum, mean, and maximum hourly heart rate (bpm) for six hourly blocks at 0:00, 6:00, 12:00, and 18:00.

	Tablet	Patch	p-Value
6:00			
Minimum	60 (55, 70.5)	60 (54.5, 68)	0.239
Mean	71 (61, 81.5)	65 (61, 76)	0.018
Maximum	85 (75, 101.5)	79 (73.5, 93)	0.003
12:00			
Minimum	66 (60.5, 73)	65 (58, 74,5)	0.615
Mean	75 (70, 87.5)	74 (68, 81.5)	0.448
Maximum	92 (83, 108.5)	89 (80.5, 105)	0.368
18:00			
Minimum	68 (61.5, 73)	66 (60.5, 72.5)	0.325
Mean	77 (67, 84.5)	72 (68, 82.5)	0.114
Maximum	91 (85.5, 101.5)	87 (77.5, 100)	0.082
0:00			
Minimum	62 (55.5, 68)	60 (55, 67.5)	0.529
Mean	67 (61, 73)	65 (58.5, 71)	0.194
Maximum	78 (69, 86.5)	76 (70, 82)	0.403

(2) We determined the total PACs and PVCs that occurred over 24 h and the PACs and PVCs per time interval (Figure 2, Table 2). Both total PACs and PVCs were significantly lower in the patch group than in the tablet group (PAC, $p = 0.015$; PVC, $p = 0.039$; Figure 2). PACs in terms of the onset per hour were not significantly different between the groups, but PVCs were significantly lower at 00:00 to 05:59 and 06:00 to 11:59 in the patch group (Table 2). Even though PVCs were observed in both groups, the majority of occurrences were isolated PVCs, and ablation therapy was not needed. In this study, mexiletine hydrochloride was orally administered for PVCs, and the dose was not modified during the study period.

(3) Systolic and diastolic blood pressure were measured at home in the early morning (Table 2), and there were no significant differences in either systolic or diastolic blood pressure measurements between the two groups.

(4) ANP and BNP levels did not change significantly over time (Table 4).

(5) Echocardiographic data showed that EF, LVDd, LVDs, E/e', and the LVMI were not significantly different between the two groups (Table 4).

Table 4. Patient echocardiographic measurements of atrial natriuretic peptide and B-type natriuretic peptide levels before and after switching from oral bisoprolol tablets to bisoprolol transdermal patch.

	0 Months (Tablet)	3 Months (Patch)	6 Months (Patch)	p-Value
ANP levels (pg/mL)	73.6 (46.9, 118.8)	65.6 (50.3, 96.1)	78.8 (45.2, 121.8)	0.341
BNP levels (pg/mL)	89.8 (41.2, 174.5)	83.4 (39.7, 174.7)	87.1 (47.9, 186.4)	0.428
Echocardiography	0 months (Tablet)		6 months (Patch)	p-value

Table 4. Cont.

	0 Months (Tablet)	3 Months (Patch)	6 Months (Patch)	p-Value
LVDd (mm)	45 (43, 51)		45 (41, 52)	0.861
LVDs (mm)	29.5 (27, 34.3)		29 (27, 34,3)	0.638
Ejection fraction (%)	64.5 (59.3, 68.3)		63.7 (59.9, 67.4)	0.400
E/e'	10,7 (7.9, 17.1)		11 (8.1, 17.3)	0.369
LVMI (g/m^2)	158.8 (121.5, 181.7)		141.1 (120.8, 164.9)	0.064

ANP: atrial natriuretic peptide, BNP: B-type natriuretic peptide, LVDd: left ventricular end-diastolic diameter, LVDs: left ventricular end-systolic diameter, E/e': the ratio of early diastolic mitral inflow to mitral annular tissue velocities, LVMI: left ventricular mass index.

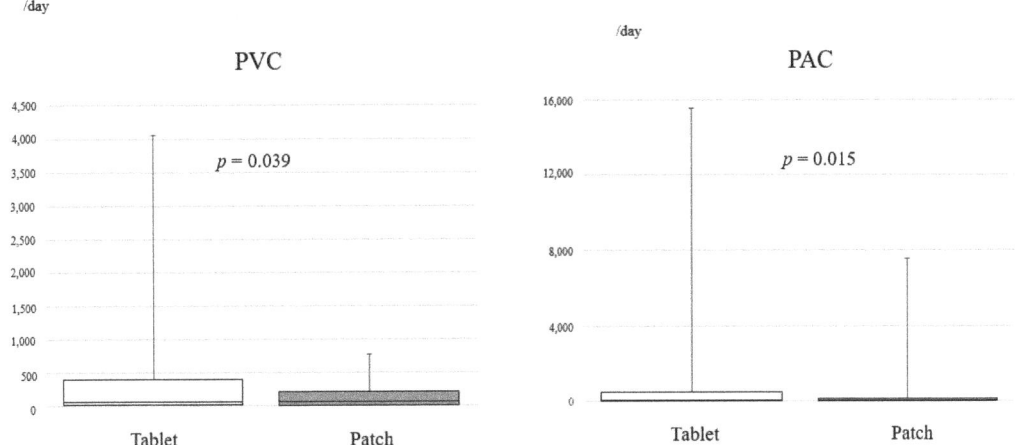

Figure 2. Bar graph showing the total number of premature ventricular contractions and premature atrial contractions over 24 h in patients from the oral bisoprolol tablet group and the bisoprolol transdermal patch group. PVCs, premature ventricular contractions; PACs, premature atrial contractions.

4. Discussion

This study indicated that the patch group had significantly lower HRs in the early morning. The total number of PACs and PVCs in 24 h was significantly lower in the patch group than in the tablet group, and the number of PVCs was significantly lower during sleep and in the morning in the patch group. With regard to the onset of arrythmia, significantly fewer PACs and PVCs occurred over 24 h in the patch group than in the tablet group, and the number of PVCs were significantly lower during sleep and in the morning in the patch group. We selected 06:00 as the study time point because cardiovascular events and sudden death are more likely to occur in the morning and during sleep. The study result shows that the effects of the patch formulation of beta-blockers last longer than those of the tablet formulation. However, it is not investigated in patients who require treatment for arrhythmia or tachycardia. As such, it is necessary to study the effects of both drug formulations in patients who need to be treated for arrhythmia or tachycardia.

In a previous study, we reported that the peak blood bisoprolol concentration after 2 weeks of treatment was 2.2 ± 0.8 h in the tablet group and 7.8 ± 2.0 h in the patch group and that the half-life was 10.02 ± 1.29 h in the tablet group and 20.80 ± 4.48 h in the patch group [6]. Blood bisoprolol concentrations were higher in the tablet group in the first 6 h after administration of the medication, and thereafter, the patch group had higher blood bisoprolol concentrations from 6 to 36 h after administration of the medication. In the present study, we did not measure the blood concentration of bisoprolol; however, because the half-life of the patch formulation is longer and the blood bisoprolol concentration from

6 to 36 h after the application is higher, we presume that the efficacy of the drug persisted during sleep and through to the morning of the next day.

Until now, only two studies have evaluated the switch from tablets to patches. Momomura et al. performed a phase II study on 40 patients with chronic heart failure who switched from oral tablets to patch formulations; the study showed favorable safety and efficacy. Based on the New York Heart Association functional classifications, there were no changes in the left ventricular functions observed by cardiac ultrasound imaging. Moreover, there were no pulse rate changes after switching to the patch. However, systolic blood pressure was significantly lower at weeks 8 and 16 after the medication switch [4]. Sairaku et al. reported that 30 patients with hypertension had their medication changed from the orally administered tablet to the patch formulation, and no differences were observed in the 24 h time domain or frequency domain of the heart rate variability (HRV) measurements. However, switching to the patch significantly altered the time-course curves of the hourly HRV measurements, which included the mean normal-to-normal (NN) interval, the standard deviation of the NN index, the high-frequency component, and the low-frequency component. Even though an equivalent dose of bisoprolol was given, the authors concluded that the autonomic modulation pattern might vary depending on whether the patient received the bisoprolol transdermally or orally [6].

To date, only two randomized studies on patients allocated to either tablet or patch versions of bisoprolol have been reported. Yamashita et al. conducted a comparative study of oral versus patch formulation in 220 patients with persistent and chronic atrial fibrillation (BBISONO-AF study). No group differences were observed in either the resting or mean HRs over 24 h measured by 12-lead ECG. They also reported that a 2.5 mg tablet is comparable to a 4 mg patch, and a 5 mg tablet is comparable to an 8 mg patch. Moreover, they found that the HR-lowering effect of the transdermal patch is most effective in the early morning when the HR is rising or when a high HR condition causes sympathetic input. Therefore, the patch was more effective in patients with sympathetic nervous tension [7]. Matsuoka et al. demonstrated that the patch had a more stable plasma concentration time profile than the tablets, and the morning heart rate was dose-dependent and significantly lower in the patch group than the tablet group [5].

Neither of these studies reported data on PVCs or PACs. However, Shinohara et al. investigated the efficacy of the bisoprolol patch by measuring the frequency of PVCs in 44 patients without structural heart disease. They reported a consistent decrease in PVC over 24 h and wrote that PVCs are triggered by sympathetic activation and that the patch formulation of bisoprolol has a longer half-life and exerts sustained effects in reducing PVCs over 24 h [8].

Concerning adverse effects, skin rash was observed in four patients in the present study. Initially, the patch was manufactured with a rubber adhesive, but an acrylic adhesive started to be used in January 2019. In this study, 23 patients used rubber adhesive patches only, 16 patients used acrylic adhesive patches only, and 11 patients used rubber adhesive patches at first and then switched to acrylic adhesive patches. Skin rash was observed in three patients (8.85%) with a rubber adhesive patch and one patient (3.7%) with an acrylic adhesive patch; the difference was not significant ($p = 0.623$). However, the question of whether the type of adhesive affects the rate of skin rash may need further investigation.

In this study, the test drug, the bisoprolol transdermal patch, was administered for 6 months, which was the longest observation period reported so far. This study demonstrated stable effects over 24 h and clearly suggested that there was parasympathetic nerve inhibition throughout the day. Although there were no significant differences in the LVMI at 6 months, a decreasing trend was observed. Therefore, a longer treatment period may result in improvement and inhibition of cardiac enlargement and prognosis. Thus, an additional study with a longer observational period is necessary to better understand these results.

5. Limitations

This study has several limitations. Although it was a prospective study, it was performed at a single center with a limited number of patients. Additionally, we only investigated the effects in patients who switched from the orally administered tablet to the transdermal patch and did not evaluate patients who switched from the patch to oral tablets. In addition, the study did not measure blood concentrations of bisoprolol, and obtaining such data would help to determine the differences between the patch and oral formulations. A 2.5 mg tablet is considered to correspond to a 4 mg patch, and a 5 mg tablet to an 8 mg patch. However, because we did not measure blood concentrations during the study period, we do not know whether there is a correlation between the doses of the two formulations. Furthermore, it is difficult to conclude whether the observed effects were due to the dose or differences in the dose because of the small number of patients. Therefore, a future study with a more robust design is required.

6. Conclusions

Compared with oral bisoprolol, the bisoprolol transdermal patch lowers HR at 06:00 and inhibits arrythmia during sleep and in the morning.

Author Contributions: A.S., H.S., M.T. (Makoto Taoka), S.O. and M.T. (Masashi Tanaka) made substantial contributions to the conception and design of this work, acquisition of data, analysis, interpretation of data, and drafting the article or revising it critically for important intellectual content. They agree to be accountable for all aspects of the published work. All authors have read and agreed to the published version of the manuscript.

Funding: This research received no external funding.

Institutional Review Board Statement: This study was conducted at Sekino Hospital, which is a logistical support hospital of the Nihon University Itabashi Hospital. The study was approved by our institutional review board (reference number 20180201-1).

Informed Consent Statement: The study details were explained to the patients and families, and written informed consent was obtained.

Data Availability Statement: In principle, the data used in this study cannot be shared.

Acknowledgments: We would like to express our sincere appreciation to Kazuaki Obata, Yoshitarou Shimizu, and Sakie Kanno, Medical Technologists at Sekino Hospital, for their constructive cooperation.

Conflicts of Interest: Akira Sezai received payment for lecture fees from Bayer, Ltd.; Bristol-Myers Squibb Company, Ltd.; Chugai Pharmaceutical Company; Mitsubishi Tanabe Pharma Company; Daiichi Sankyo Company, Ltd.; and Pfizer Inc. The other authors declare no conflict of interest associated with this study.

Clinical Trial Registration: UMIN (http://www.umin.ac.jp/; accessed on 1 January 2022), study ID: UMIN000031538.

References

1. Bauersachs, J. Heart failure drug treatment: The fantastic four. *Eur. Heart J.* **2021**, *42*, 681–683. [CrossRef] [PubMed]
2. Heidenreich, P.A.; Bozkurt, B.; Aguilar, D.; Allen, L.A.; Byun, J.J.; Colvin, M.M.; Deswal, A.; Drazner, M.H.; Dunlay, S.M.; Evers, L.R.; et al. 2022 AHA/ACC/HFSA guideline for the management of heart failure: A report of the American College of Cardiology/American Heart Association joint committee on clinical practice guidelines. *J. Am. Coll. Cariol.* **2022**, *79*, e263–e421. [CrossRef] [PubMed]
3. Schnabbel, P.; Maack, C.; Mies, F.; Tyroller, S.; Scheer, A.; Böhm, M. Binding properties of beta-blockers at recombinant beta1-, beta 2, beta 3-adrenoceptors. *J. Cadiovasc. Pharmmacol.* **2000**, *36*, 466–471. [CrossRef] [PubMed]
4. Momomura, S.I.; Saito, Y.; Yasumura, Y.; Yamamoto, K.; Sakata, Y.; Daimon, M.; Kinugawa, K.; Okamoto, H.; Dohi, N.; Komuro, I. Efficacy and safety of switching from oral bisoprolol to transdermal patch in japanese patients with chronic heart failure. *Circ. J.* **2017**, *2*, 141–147. [CrossRef] [PubMed]

5. Matsuoka, H.; Kuwajima, I.; Shimada, K.; Mitamura, H.; Saruta, T. Comparison of efficacy and safety between bisoprolol transdermal patch (TY-0201) and bisoprolol fumarate oral formulation in Japanese patients with grade I or II essential hypertension: Randomized, double-blind, placebo-controlled study. *J. Clin. Hypertens.* **2013**, *15*, 806–814. [CrossRef] [PubMed]
6. Sairaku, A.; Nakano, Y.; Shiode, N.; Suennari, K.; Oda, N.; Ono, K.; Kihara, Y. Head-to-head comparison of the heart rate variability between the bisoprolol transdermal patch and bisoprolol fumarate tablet. *Cardiovasc. Ther.* **2018**, *36*, e12325. [CrossRef] [PubMed]
7. Yammashita, T.; Ikeda, T.; Akita, Y. Comparison of heart rate reduction effect and safety between bisoprolol transdermal patch and bisoprolol fumarate oral formulation in Japanese patients with persistent/permanent atrial fibrillation (BISONO-AF study). *J. Cardiol.* **2019**, *3*, 386–393. [CrossRef] [PubMed]
8. Shinohara, M.; Fujino, T.; Yao, S.; Yano, K.; Akitsu, K.; Koike, H.; Yuzawa, H.Y.; Suzuki, T.S.; Fukunaga, S.F.; Kobayashi, K.K.; et al. Assessment of a novel transdermal selective b1-blocker, the bisoprolol patch, for treating frequent premature ventricular contractions in patients without structural heart disease. *J. Cardiol.* **2019**, *73*, 7–13. [CrossRef] [PubMed]

Disclaimer/Publisher's Note: The statements, opinions and data contained in all publications are solely those of the individual author(s) and contributor(s) and not of MDPI and/or the editor(s). MDPI and/or the editor(s) disclaim responsibility for any injury to people or property resulting from any ideas, methods, instructions or products referred to in the content.

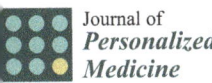

Article

Positivity and Health Locus of Control: Key Variables to Intervene on Well-Being of Cardiovascular Disease Patients

Bárbara Luque [1,2], Naima Z. Farhane-Medina [1,2], Marta Villalba [2], Rosario Castillo-Mayén [1,2,*], Esther Cuadrado [1,2] and Carmen Tabernero [1,3,4]

1. Maimonides Biomedical Research Institute of Cordoba (IMIBIC), 14004 Córdoba, Spain; bluque@uco.es (B.L.); z62famen@uco.es (N.Z.F.-M.); esther.cuadrado@uco.es (E.C.); carmen.tabernero@usal.es (C.T.)
2. Department of Psychology, University of Cordoba, 14071 Cordoba, Spain
3. Institute of Neurosciences of Castilla y León (INCYL), University of Salamanca, 37007 Salamanca, Spain
4. Department of Social Psychology and Anthropology, University of Salamanca, 37005 Salamanca, Spain
* Correspondence: rcmayen@uco.es

Abstract: Psychological well-being is a good predictor of several health outcomes in cardiovascular disease patients (adherence, quality of life, and healthy behaviors). The perception of health control and a positive orientation seem to have a beneficial effect on health and well-being. Therefore, the aim of this study was to investigate the role of the health locus of control and positivity in the psychological well-being and quality of life of cardiovascular patients. A total of 593 cardiac outpatients completed the Multidimensional Health Locus of Control Scale, the Positivity Scale and the Hospital Anxiety and Depression Scale at baseline (January 2017) and 9 m later (follow-up; n = 323). A Spearman rank correlation coefficient and a structural equation modeling approach were determined to explore the relationships between those variables both cross-sectionally and longitudinally. A cross-sectional correlation analysis at baseline revealed that the internal health locus of control and positivity were negatively associated with anxiety (r_s = −0.15 and −0.44, ps < 0.01) and depression (r_s = −0.22 and −0.55, ps < 0.01) and positively associated with health-related quality of life (r_s = 0.16 and 0.46, ps < 0.01). Similar outcomes were found at follow-up and in longitudinal correlations. According to the path analysis, positivity was found to be negatively associated with anxiety and depression level at baseline (β = −0.42 and −0.45, ps < 0.001). Longitudinally, positivity was negatively associated with depression (β = 0.15, p < 0.01) and together with the internal health locus of control, was positively associated with health-related quality of life (β = 0.16 and 0.10, respectively, ps < 0.05). These findings suggest that focusing on the health locus of control and especially positivity may be crucial in enhancing the psychological well-being of patients in the context of cardiac care. The potential impact of these results on future interventions is discussed.

Keywords: cardiovascular disease (CVD); health locus of control; positivity; psychological well-being; health-related quality of life

1. Introduction

Cardiovascular disease (CVD) is a broad term that encompasses various medical conditions affecting the heart and blood vessels [1]. These conditions include coronary artery disease, heart failure, arrhythmias, valvular heart disease, and peripheral artery disease, among others [1]. CVD is highly prevalent worldwide, and this trend appears to be increasing. Recent data from the Global Burden of Cardiovascular Diseases and Risk Factors [2] show that the total prevalence of CVD has nearly doubled in the last three decades, from 271 million in 1990 to 523 million in 2019. The increase in prevalence has been accompanied by a significant rise in disability-adjusted life years and years lived with disability from 17.1 million to 34.4 in the same period, as well as an alarming mortality rate among affected patients [2]. With its different typologies, CVD remains the leading cause of death worldwide [3]. To such an extent that according to the World Health Organization [4], in 2019, 17.9 million people died due to CVD, representing 32% of global deaths. The enormous burden of this health condition [5] has led to the need for working at a preventive level, from health promotion to the implementation of interventions that reduce associated risk factors [6]. This aspect has become a real challenge for healthcare systems from all disciplines that address these types of diseases [7,8].

There are several risk factors related to CVD, but psychosocial factors are particularly relevant due to their influence in this disease [6,7,9]. According to the European Society of Cardiology [10], some of the psychosocial risk factors noted are low socio-economic status, lack of social support, Type D personality, stress at work and in family life, hostility, depression, and anxiety [9]. Therefore, from a biopsychosocial approach of health, interventions for CVD patients should also address their psychological well-being to mitigate the emotional consequences of the diagnosis [6,8,11]. To design effective integrative interventions for CVD patients, it is crucial to explore which psychological variables influence cardiovascular health (CVH) and well-being, as well as the role of personality dispositions in these variables. This approach could be beneficial both in the prevention and treatment of CVD, considering individual differences in psychological profiles [12,13]. For these reasons, incorporating a psychosocial approach in cardiac rehabilitation could improve the clinical management of CVD and have a positive impact on patient outcomes [14].

1.1. CVD and Psychological Well-Being and Quality of Life

Psychological well-being is a complex term to define, but it is typically associated with positive thoughts and emotions that individuals experience regarding their life satisfaction and overall sense of worth [15]. Therefore, it refers to optimal psychological functioning, which includes a combination of emotional aspects (e.g., happiness and experiencing positive emotions) as well as higher-level functions such as resilience, coping, and emotional regulation [15,16]. In contrast, psychological distress is composed of constructs such as anxiety, depression, anguish, or hostility [17].

Recent research has shown the association and relevance of psychological well-being or distress among patients with CVD [11,18,19]. Studies have found that increased levels of well-being were related to improved CVH [11] and lower odds of mortality due to a cardiac event [6,20]. Conversely, psychological distress, specifically depression and anxiety, has been bidirectionally linked to CVD [9,21]. Meta-analyses and longitudinal studies have provided evidence that depression and anxiety are risk factors for CVD, with an association between them and an increased risk of developing heart diseases such as ischemic heart disease or coronary heart disease [22–24]. In addition, the diagnosis of CVD may exacerbate anxiety and depressive symptoms in these patients. Some studies have reported a high prevalence of depression among patients with coronary artery disease, with 34% of them experiencing moderate to severe depression, which could negatively affect their prognosis [25]. A meta-analysis performed by Gathright et al. [26] found that depression was a predictor of all-cause mortality in heart failure. Furthermore, patients with coronary heart disease or heart failure and depressive symptoms are more likely to have a lower quality of life and a greater risk for recurrent cardiovascular events and mortality [23]. At the same time, studies addressing psychological distress and CVD have showed some sex differences. Women with CVD reported greater and more severe symptomatology of anxiety and depression than men with CVD [27,28], highlighting the need to consider these differences when designing and applying treatments for CVD patients.

CVD can have a significant impact on patients' lives, not only causing psychological distress mentioned above but also physical symptoms such as reduced mobility, pain, and fatigue [29]. These symptoms may become chronic and can negatively affect their quality of life [13]. Previous studies have shown the association between a CVD diagnosis and a lower HRQoL [30,31], which includes physical, mental, and social factors, as well as subjective perceptions of health and well-being [32]. At the same time, lower HRQoL is associated with other CVD risk factors such as a reduced adherence to medication and an in-creased risk of recurrent cardiovascular events [33–35]. These findings have led to a wide body of research studying the role of HRQoL as an important variable in the context of chronic conditions, such as CVD, in order to better understand and intervene on its impact.

The impact of psychological distress on the quality of life of individuals with cardiovascular disease emphasizes the need to intervene in their emotional and psychological care [6–9,14]. Further research is necessary to identify key variables that promote their psychological well-being and provide protective effects against the disease.

1.2. CVD and Personality Dispositions: Positivity and Health Locus of Control

Personality dispositions are consistent patterns of thoughts, feelings, and behaviors that characterizes an individual and are relatively stable over time and across different contexts [36]. Some personality dispositions have been found to be related to well-being and quality of life, such as positivity and the health locus of control (HLC). Positivity is a psychological construct that provides insights into individuals' overall sense of wellness as it can be defined by factors such as self-esteem, satisfaction with life, and optimism [37]—factors that have been studied by their association with chronic conditions. For instance, self-esteem has been found to mediate the relationship between life satisfaction and lower depression in CVD patients [38]. Optimism, on the other hand, seems to favor other psychological and cognitive mechanisms that promote better cardiovascular health (CVH) [11,18,39], reduce the risk of cardiovascular events [40], and facilitate the engaging of health-related behaviors [39]. In addition, several studies have found that positivity is a significant predictor of psychological variables related to psychological well-being and quality of life, such as depression and anxiety [11,37,41], as well as to the prognosis of the disease, reducing the rate of rehospitalization and mortality [41]. Therefore, encouraging individuals to adopt a more positive outlook on life, including their illness, would be necessary to help them feel more in control and self-efficacious in coping with their situation [18,40]. Thus, another much related and equally important variable would be the health locus of control.

Improving a CVH prognosis involves making lifestyle changes [42], which can be influenced by various factors, including the personality disposition of HLC [43]. HLC refers to people's beliefs about their ability to control their health, which can be either internal or external [43]. Internal HLC refers to individuals' perception of having control over their health, while external HLC refers to the belief that external factors, such as genetics, chance, or other people including family and physicians, have control over one's health [44]. According to the Health Locus of Control Theory, individuals' health-related behaviors are associated with their perception of their ability to overcome health problems. Internal HLC has been found to be linked to engage in positive and protective health behaviors [45,46]. On the other hand, individuals with external HLC may have a lower sense of personal responsibility for one's own health, which may result in worse health outcomes and a poorer disease prognosis [47].

The literature shows the significant role of psychological variables and personality traits in better understanding and conceptualizing the onset and consequences of CVD in a person's life. However, there is still a need to further investigate the specific mechanisms that underlie the association between these variables. Such research could provide valuable information for designing future psychological treatments and enhancing the effectiveness of cardiac rehabilitation programs, leading to improved psychological well-being and quality of life for CVD patients.

1.3. Aim and Hypotheses

The aim of this research was to explore the influence of HLC and positivity variables on psychological well-being, considering levels of anxiety and depression, and HRQoL in patients with CVD over time. For this purpose, the evaluations of these variables were carried out at two different times, thus being able to obtain results of the same variables in a first phase (baseline), and after approximately 9 months in a second phase (follow-up). The hypotheses proposed for this study were as follows (Figure 1):

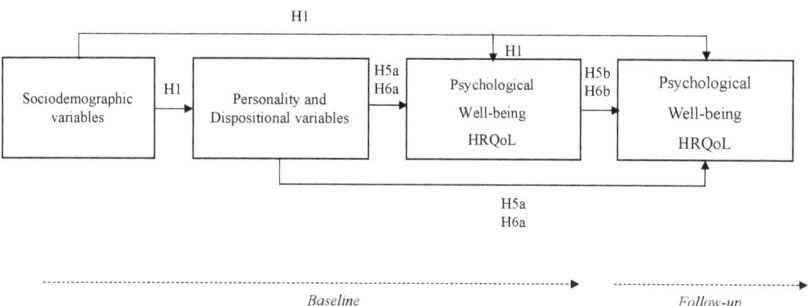

Figure 1. Proposed research hypothesis model. Sociodemographic variables: age, sex, economic and educational level, etc. Personality and dispositional variables: positivity and health locus of control. Psychological well-being: levels of anxiety and depression; HRQoL: health-related quality of life. The model does not include H2, H3, and H4 as they refer to correlations between variables rather than predictive relationships.

Hypothesis H1. *Sociodemographic variables are significantly associated with the dispositional variables, psychological well-being and the HRQoL.*

Hypothesis H2. *Patients with higher levels of positivity will have lower levels of anxiety and depression, and therefore greater psychological well-being as well as higher health-related quality of life, both cross-sectionally (H2a) and longitudinally (H2b).*

Hypothesis H3. *The patients with higher levels of internal HLC will have lower levels of anxiety and depression, and therefore greater psychological well-being and HRQoL, both cross-sectionally (H3a) and longitudinally (H3b).*

Hypothesis H4. *The internal HLC and positivity, given the stability of personality dispositions, will maintain similar correlations with psychological well-being and HRQoL both at baseline and at follow-up.*

Hypothesis H5. *Positivity will predict the levels of psychological well-being and HRQoL variables (dependent variables) in patients, both cross-sectionally (H5a) and longitudinally (H5b).*

Hypothesis H6. *The internal HLC will predict the levels of psychological well-being and HRQoL variables (dependent variables) in patients, both cross-sectionally (H6a) and longitudinally (H6b).*

2. Materials and Methods

2.1. Participants and Procedure

This study included 593 CVD patients ($M = 64.75$, $SD = 9.07$) recruited from the Cardiology Unit of the University Reina Sofía Hospital (Córdoba, Spain) who participated in the CORDIOPREV study [48,49] using a convenience sampling method. The inclusion and exclusion criteria of this study followed those of the primary study. Patients that had already suffered a first cardiac event and were diagnosed with an established coronary heart disease (e.g., unstable coronary disease, acute myocardial infarction, chronic coronary disease, and unstable angina) were included. CVD patients that had experienced a clinical event in the last 6 months were excluded. The study sample characteristics had been previously published [48,49].

A longitudinal study was designed to test the hypotheses proposed. A battery of questionnaires was administered to the participants to assess HLC, positivity, psychological well-being through the components of anxiety and depression, and HRQoL at two different times. The baseline assessment started in January 2017 and the follow-up evaluation was conducted approximately 9 months later. At baseline, the sample was composed of 593 patients, and at follow-up of 323 CVD patients. Sociodemographic characteristics measured are shown in Table 1.

Table 1. Patients' sociodemographic characteristics (n = 593).

Sociodemographic Characteristics		Frequencies	(%)
Sex			
	Male	508	85.7
	Female	85	14.3
Age, Mean (SD) = 64.75 (9.07)			
Employment status			
	Unemployed	29	4.9
	Part-time worker	17	2.9
	Full-time worker	119	20.1
	Retired	398	67.1
	Housework	30	5.1
Partner			
	Yes/With	527	88.9
	No/Without	66	11.1
Educational level			
	Very low	1	0.2
	Low	18	3.0
	Middle	332	56.0
	High	226	38.1
	Very high	16	2.7
Economic level			
	Very low	8	1.3
	Low	90	15.2
	Middle	460	77.6
	High	35	5.9

The current study was approved by the corresponding Research Ethics Committees (June 2015). Prior to their participation, all patients were informed about this study's objectives and assured that their involvement would be voluntary and anonymous. Those who consented to participate provided written informed consent. Participants completed the questionnaires using tablets in a designated room at the hospital. The surveys were conducted using the Unipark program (v. 10.9), which is an online survey software available through the Questback academic program. Sociodemographic characteristics measured are shown in Table 1.

2.2. Instruments

Sociodemographic ad hoc questionnaire. The study participants were asked to provide sociodemographic details such as their sex, age, employment status, marital status (whether they had a partner), educational background, and economic status.

Multidimensional Health Locus of Control Scale (MHLC-S [46]). The MHLC-S evaluates the locus of control for health. It is composed of four factors according to whom the control is assigned, which in this study are termed: internal HLC; chance HLC; doctors HLC; and other people HLC. Although the original scale contains 24 items (e.g., "*I am directly responsible for my condition getting better or worse*"), in this study, a short version of the scale composed of 12 items was used (each factor contains 3 items). It uses a Likert response format of 7 points in a range of 1 (strongly disagree) to 7 (strongly agree). The original study shows a measure with Cronbach's alpha between 0.66 and 0.77. Due to the low reliability of the doctor's factor in this study, it was excluded from the analysis. However, after deleting this subscale, Confirmatory Factor Analyses indicated a good model fit of the scale at both measurement moments. The fit indices at T1 were: $\chi^2 (24) = 84.86$, $p < 0.001$; RMSEA (90% CI) = 0.07 (0.05, 0.08); CFI = 0.96; TLI = 0.95; GFI = 0.97; and AGFI = 0.94. At T2, the fit indices were $\chi^2(21) = 49.59$, $p = 0.002$; RMSEA (90% CI) = 0.06 (0.04, 0.08); CFI = 0.97; TLI = 0.96; GFI = 0.97; and AGFI = 0.93.

Positivity Scale (P-scale [37]). This scale evaluates the personal tendency to interpret life and vital experiences from a positive point of view. It is a unidimensional scale that contains eight items (e.g., "*I have great faith in the future*") ranging from 1 (*strongly disagree*) to 5 (*strongly agree*). A higher score indicates greater positivity. Previous studies have reported adequate internal consistency of the measure in different countries, including Spain, with a Cronbach's alpha of 0.81 [37].

Hospital Anxiety and Depression Scale (HADS [50], Spanish validation from Terol et al. [51]). The HADS is a self-administered scale that allows the evaluation of psychological well-being considering the total score on the scale, as well as from the two factors that compose it: anxiety (HADS-A; e.g., "*I get sort of a frightened feeling as if something awful is about to happen*") and depression (HADS-D; e.g., "*I feel as if I am slowed down*"). This measure is composed of 14 items distributed in anxiety and depression subscales, each one having 7 items and with a 7-point frequency scale ranging from 1 (*never*) to 7 (*every day*). A higher score indicates higher levels of anxiety and depression, respectively, and therefore a lower level of psychological well-being when considering the total score of the scale. Previous studies have reported adequate internal consistency: $\alpha = 0.78$ in HADS-A, $\alpha = 0.82$ in HADS-D, and $\alpha = 0.89$ in the general scale [51].

The *Short Form-12 Health Survey* (SF-12 [52], Spanish validation from Failde et al. [53]). The SF-12 is a self-report questionnaire that assesses health-related quality of life. It consists of 12 items that measure 8 domains related to health: physical functioning, role limitations due to physical problems, bodily pain, general health perceptions, vitality, social functioning, role limitations due to emotional problems, and mental health. These domains are subdivided in a mental health component (MCS; six items: e.g., "*have you had any problems with your work or other regular daily activities as a result of your emotional problem (such as feeling depressed or anxious)?*") and a physical health component (PCS; six items: e.g., "*Does your health now limit you in walking several blocks?*"). From the twelve items, eight were presented on a 5-point Likert-type scale and four in a dichotomous format that required a 'yes' or 'no' response. Higher scores indicate better health-related quality of life. Previous studies have reported adequate internal consistency: $\alpha = 0.85$ in PCS and $\alpha = 0.78$ in MCS [54].

2.3. Statistical Analysis

Descriptive statistics were conducted to know the frequencies of the sociodemographic characteristics. Subsequently, a Kolmogorov–Smirnov test was conducted to determine whether the data were normally distributed. The results conclude that the assumption of normality was violated in all evaluated scales. Therefore, we performed Spearman's rank correlation analyses to measure the association between the variables cross-sectionally and longitudinally. Then, we conducted a path analysis using the structural equation modelling (SEM) approach to further explore the explanatory capacity of the HLC and positivity on psychological well-being, anxiety and depression factors, and health-related quality of life. The model's adequacy was evaluated by means of several metrics, including the chi-squared statistic (χ^2), the comparative fit index (CFI), the Tucker–Lewis index (TLI), the root mean square error of approximation (RMSEA), and the standardized root mean square residual (SRMR). For model evaluation, we followed the recommendations of Schermelleh-Engel et al. [55]. According to these authors, an acceptable model fit is indicated by a χ^2/df value that is equal to or less than 3, as well as CFI and NNFI values that are equal to or greater than 0.95, and RMSEA values that are less than 0.08, accompanied by a confidence interval (CI) that is in close proximity to RMSEA. The independent variables were "health locus of control (HLC)" and "positivity", while the dependent variables were "psychological well-being" assessed through levels of "anxiety" and "depression", and HRQoL. A descriptive analysis and Spearman's correlations were performed using the statistic software SPSS (v.28) and to estimate the path coefficients, we used the software package AMOS (v.13). To interpret correlation results, we considered Cohen's (1988) [56] suggestions, where a correlation coefficient of 0.1 to 0.3 was considered small, 0.3 to 0.5 was moderate, and greater than 0.5 was large. For both analyses, we set the significance level at $p < 0.05$.

3. Results

3.1. Sociodemographic Characteristics of Participants

Sociodemographic features of the participants are presented in Table 1. The study sample was majorly composed of men [85.7%]. Regarding labor status, most of the participants were retired [67.1%], followed by having a full-time job [20.1%], houseworkers [5.1%], unemployed [4.9%], and part-time workers [2.9%]. Regarding marital status, most patients had a partner [88.9%]. Finally, the highest number of respondents had received middle educational qualification [56%], followed by high educational level [38.1%], low [3%], very high [2.7%], and very low [0.2%].

3.2. Cross-Sectional Analysis

In the first correlation analysis, data were obtained on the associations between all variables (at baseline and at follow-up independently). The significant correlations between the study variables were as follows (Table 2): at baseline, the other people HLC correlated negatively with depression ($r_s = -0.22$) as well as with psychological distress ($r_s = -0.17$); the internal HLC correlated negatively with anxiety ($r_s = -0.15$) and depression ($r_s = -0.22$) and with psychological distress ($r_s = -0.20$) and positively with all the HRQoL (global, $r_s = 0.16$; MCS, $r_s = 0.14$; PCS, $r_s = 0.15$). Moreover, the internal HLC was positively associated with the other people HLC factor ($r_s = 0.26$) and positivity ($r_s = 0.13$); the chance HLC correlated negatively with depression only ($r_s = -0.10$). Finally, positivity correlated positively with the internal and other people HLC ($r_s = 0.13$, $r_s = 0.20$, respectively) and all HRQoL factors (global, $r_s = 0.46$; MCS, $r_s = 0.51$; PCS, $r_s = 0.34$), and negatively with psychological distress ($r_s = -0.55$), depression ($r_s = -0.55$), and anxiety ($r_s = -0.44$). At follow-up, the only differences were that the internal HLC did not positively correlate with the PCS HRQoL. Other people HLC correlated negatively with anxiety ($r_s = -0.19$) and positively with MCS HRQoL ($r_s = 0.16$). Thus, most of the correlation results remained stable over time.

3.3. Longitudinal Analysis

The second correlation analysis was conducted to identify any statistically significant relationships between the evaluated variables at baseline and at follow-up (Table 3). Regarding the independent variables, the three HLC factors at baseline significantly correlated with themselves at follow-up (internal HLC, $r_s = 0.44$; other people HLC, $r_s = 0.47$; and chance HLC, $r_s = 0.43$). Only other people HLC was significantly associated with positivity at follow-up ($r_s = 0.18$). In contrast, baseline positivity correlated with the variables' positivity ($r_s = 0.54$), other people HLC ($r_s = 0.23$), and internal HLC ($r_s = 0.17$) at follow-up. On the other hand, with respect to the association between independent and dependent variables, several significant data were found. Baseline scores of the other people HLC correlated negatively with follow-up psychological distress ($r_s = -0.17$), anxiety ($r_s = -0.13$), depression ($r_s = -0.22$), and PCS HRQoL ($r_s = -0.14$); the internal HLC showed similar outcomes, but with the difference that this factor correlated positively with the global ($r_s = 0.13$) and MCS HRQoL ($r_s = 0.16$) and not with the PCS HRQoL and anxiety; the chance HLC did not correlate significantly with any dependent variable. Finally, baseline positivity correlated negatively with follow-up anxiety ($r_s = -0.35$), depression ($r_s = -0.36$), and psychological distress ($r_s = -0.39$) and positively with all HRQoL factors (global, $r_s = 0.33$; MCS, $r_s = 0.36$; PCS, $r_s = 0.26$).

Table 2. Cross-sectional correlation analysis of all variables at baseline (a) and at follow-up (b).

(a)	Baseline (n = 593)									
	1	2	3	4	5	6	7	8	9	10
1. Other people HLC	1									
2. Internal HLC	0.26 **	1								
3. Chance HLC	0.30 **	−0.02	1							
4. Positivity	0.20 **	0.13 **	0.07	1						
5. HADS	−0.17 **	−0.20 **	−0.05	−0.55 **	1					
6. Anxiety	−0.09	−0.15 **	−0.02	−0.44 **	0.91 **	1				
7. Depression	−0.22 **	−0.22 **	−0.10 *	−0.55 **	0.86 **	0.58 **	1			
8. SF-12	−0.02	0.16 **	−0.02	0.46 **	−0.63 **	−0.54 **	−0.59 **	1		
9. SF-12 (MCS)	0.05	0.14 **	0.01	0.51 **	−0.73 **	−0.65 **	−0.65 **	−0.88 *	1	
10. SF-12 (PCS)	−0.03	0.15 **	−0.06	0.34 **	−0.43 **	−0.38 **	−0.44 **	−0.91 **	0.61 **	1

(b)	Follow-up (n = 323)									
	1	2	3	4	5	6	7	8	9	10
1. Other people HLC	1									
2. Internal HLC	0.25 **	1								
3. Chance HLC	0.39 **	0.05	1							
4. Positivity	0.29 **	0.15 **	0.10	1						
5. HADS	−0.29 **	−0.25 **	−0.11	−0.48 **	1					
6. Anxiety	−0.19 *	−0.21 *	−0.06	−0.43 **	0.93 **	1				
7. Depression	−0.36 **	−0.27 **	−0.19 **	−0.47 **	0.86 **	0.64 **	1			
8. SF-12	0.10	0.15 **	−0.01	0.39 **	−0.56 **	−0.53 **	−0.47 **	1		
9. SF-12 (MCS)	0.16 **	0.18 **	−0.02	0.44 **	−0.67 **	−0.65 **	−0.54 **	0.87 **	1	
10. SF-12 (PCS)	0.04	0.09	0.00	0.29 **	−0.38 **	−0.33 **	−0.34 **	0.91 **	0.61 **	1

Note. HLC = health locus of control; HADS = Hospital Anxiety and Depression Scale; MCS = mental component summary; PCS = physical component summary; SF-12 = Short Form-12 Health Survey; * $p < 0.05$; ** $p < 0.01$.

Table 3. Longitudinal correlation analysis of all variables.

	Follow-Up (n = 323)									
Baseline	1	2	3	4	5	6	7	8	9	10
1. Other people HLC	0.47 **	0.24 **	0.22 **	0.18 **	−0.17 **	−0.13 **	−0.22 **	−0.06	0.05	−0.14 *
2. Internal HLC	0.22 **	0.44 **	−0.10	0.10	−0.14 *	−0.09	−0.16 **	0.13 *	0.16 **	0.08
3. Chance HLC	0.19 **	−0.01	0.43 **	0.04	−0.03	0.01	−0.06	−0.09	−0.08	−0.08
4. Positivity	0.23 **	0.17 **	0.02	0.54 **	−0.39 **	−0.35 **	−0.36 **	0.33 **	0.36 **	0.26 **
5. HADS	−0.24 **	−0.16 **	−0.04	−0.41 **	0.60 **	0.58 **	0.50 **	−0.35 **	−0.44 **	−0.22 **
6. Anxiety	−0.14 *	−0.13 *	0.00	−0.32 **	0.55 **	0.58 **	0.39 **	−0.31 **	−0.41 **	−0.16 **
7. Depression	−0.29 **	−0.19 **	−0.10	−0.43 **	0.51 **	0.41 **	0.54 **	−0.32 **	−0.37 **	−0.23 **
8. SF-12	0.12 *	0.06	−0.07	0.33 **	−0.45 **	−0.39 **	−0.39 **	−0.60 **	0.53 **	0.54 **
9. SF-12 (MCS)	0.18 **	0.09	−0.02	0.36 **	−0.51 **	−0.47 **	−0.44 **	0.49 **	0.55 **	0.36 **
10. SF-12 (PCS)	0.04	0.00	−0.11	0.23 **	−0.29 **	−0.22 **	−0.27 **	0.54 **	0.39 **	0.57 **

Note. HLC = health locus of control; HADS = Hospital Anxiety and Depression Scale; MCS = mental component summary; PCS = physical component summary; SF-12 = Short Form-12 Health Survey; * $p < 0.05$; ** $p < 0.01$.

After performing correlation analyses, it was observed that the diagonal, i.e., the variables (dependent and independent) at baseline, correlated positively with themselves with a mostly large magnitude [56] at follow-up. Additionally, associations were found between the independent and dependent variables in these correlations (Table 3). Based on these findings, further comprehensive evaluations were conducted to examine the predictive potential of positivity and HLC variables on psychological well-being, anxiety, depression, and HRQoL both cross-sectionally and longitudinally. To achieve this, a path analysis was performed. The model (Figure 1) demonstrated a strong fit to the data, with the following indices: $\chi2$ (37, n = 323) = 41.636, p = 0.276; CMIN/DF = 1.125; CFI = 0.995; TLI = 0.991; AGFI = 0.957, GFI = 0.980, RMSEA = 0.020, 95% CI [0.001, 0.046]). Figure 2 displays the standardized parameter estimates.

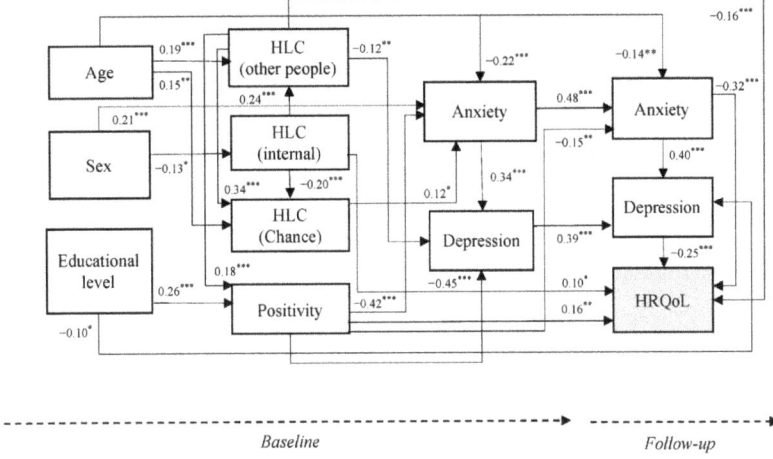

Figure 2. Standardized model parameter estimates (* p < 0.05; ** p < 0.01; *** p < 0.001). HLC = health locus of control; HRQoL = health-related quality of life. The figure only shows significant paths (n = 323).

As it can be seen in Figure 2, at baseline, positivity was negatively related to anxiety (β = −0.42, p < 0.001) and depression (β = −0.45, p < 0.001). The internal HLC was positively related to the other people HLC (β = 0.24, p < 0.001), and negatively with chance HLC (β = −0.20, p < 0.001) but not with the dependent variables. Other people HLC was negatively related to depression (β = −0.12, p < 0.01). At follow-up, no significant relationship was found between the independent (positivity and HLC) and dependent variables (anxiety, depression, and HRQoL). Longitudinally, positivity negatively predicted anxiety (β = −0.15, p < 0.01) and positively the global HRQoL (β = 0.16, p < 0.01). The internal and other people HLC also predicted the global HRQoL positively (β = 0.10, p < 0.05) and negatively (β = −0.16, p < 0.001), respectively.

Besides these associations, other relationships between dependent variables both cross-sectionally and longitudinally were also found. For instance, anxiety and depression at baseline positively predicted anxiety (β = 0.48, p < 0.001) and depression (β = 0.39, p < 0.001) at follow-up, respectively. Cross-sectionally, at follow-up, anxiety was positively related to depression (β = 0.40, p < 0.001) and both anxiety and depression were negatively related to the global HRQoL (β = −0.32 and −0.25, respectively, both ps < 0.001).

Finally, the results of the path analysis showed some significant associations between the sociodemographic variables age, sex, and educational level that need to be acknowledged. Being female was associated with higher levels of anxiety (β = 0.21, p < 0.001) and lower levels of internal HLC (β = −0.13, p < 0.05). Age was positively associated with other people (β = 0.19, p < 0.001) and chance HLC (β = 0.15, p < 0.01), and negatively with anxiety both at baseline (β = −0.22, p < 0.001) and at follow-up (β = −0.14, p < 0.01). Finally, the educational level was positively related to positivity at baseline (β = 0.26, p < 0.001) and to lower levels of depression at follow-up (β = −0.10, p < 0.01).

4. Discussion

The aim of this study was to analyze the influence of HLC and positivity on the general psychological well-being, based on the levels of anxiety and depression, and HRQoL of patients with CVD. The results found were in line with what was hypothesized in H2a and H3a. Both positivity and internal HLC correlated significantly and negatively with the dependent variables, anxiety and depression, and positively with psychological well-being and HRQoL, both at baseline and at follow-up. With respect to H2b, the results were also as expected since positivity still showed the same significant relationships with the dependent variables after 9 months (longitudinal correlation). The study's findings were also in line with H3b because internal HLC correlated positively with psychological well-being and HRQoL factors (except PCS) and negatively with depression; however, there was no significant relationship with anxiety. Furthermore, it should be noted that the factor of other people HLC showed similar associations to the internal HLC regarding the dependent variables, proving to be more related to the well-being of patients with CVD than anticipated. Finally, the results of the correlation analysis supported H4. The personality dispositions of internal HLC and positivity maintained similar correlations with anxiety, depression, and HRQoL at both assessment points, indicating consistent and stable associations between the analyzed variables.

With respect to H5a and H6a, the results partially support the hypotheses. Specifically, positivity predicted psychological well-being at baseline, but not at follow-up. Additionally, no significant results were found between internal HLC and the other dependent variables, neither at baseline nor at follow-up. As expected, the relationship between the independent variables, positivity in this case, with the dependent variables was negative. This means that higher levels of positivity corresponded to lower levels of anxiety, depression, and psychological discomfort, ultimately leading to greater well-being. These findings align with previous research, underscoring the significance of positivity in the psychological well-being of CVD patients [11,18,19]. Maintaining a positive outlook can help prevent emotional states that may become pathological when prolonged, such as elevated levels of anxiety and depression. Improved psychological well-being may, in turn, lead to a better prognosis for CVD patients. Results such as those obtained in the meta-analysis of DuBois et al. [41] have shown the association of positive emotions with the reduction of mortality in CVD, which is another sign that these emotions benefit psychological well-being and therefore a cardiovascular prognosis. Alessandri et al. [57] stated in their work that positivity acted as a variable that promotes positive affect (this being a component of subjective well-being) and serves as a buffer for depression and negative affect. The introduction of the present study mentioned the importance of optimism, which is one of the components of positivity. Some studies, such as Sahoo et al. [58], highlighted the protective role of personality traits such as optimism against the development of CVD; similarly, others argued that a higher level of optimism led to a lower risk of CVD mortality and lower levels of anxiety and depression [59].

Regarding H5b, the results of this study partially support this hypothesis, which suggests that positivity has the potential to predict lower levels of anxiety and higher levels of HRQoL over time. The findings provide further evidence of the significance of positivity, not only for its influence on emotional aspects at specific moments but also for its long-term impact, in line with previous studies [60]. These results indicate that positivity may be a useful tool for improving patient outcomes and highlight the need for further research on this construct as an intervention for CVD patients, given its potential to positively impact their long-term health and well-being.

Finally, H6b is also partially supported by the findings of this study. However, considering the importance of the internal HLC manifested in the literature, it was anticipated that this variable would be a strong predictor across all dependent variables over time. Nevertheless, the capacity of prediction was only found related to HRQoL. Although different from what was expected, these results demonstrate a significant approach to the subject. Firstly, this study's results align with previous research that outlines the association between internal

HLC and HRQoL in CVD patients [47,61]. The influence of internal HLC on the quality of life of CVD patients has also been demonstrated by its impact on modifiable risk factors. Internal HLC has been associated with increased physical activity dedication, decreased alcohol consumption, and even lower mortality rates among cardiac patients [61,62]. Furthermore, internal HLC has been linked to various health-related outcomes associated to HRQoL in chronic patients. For instance, it has been shown to promote better maintenance of physical function after hospitalization [63], increase resilience, reduce stress, enhance physical activity and lower drug consumption among patients with pain conditions [64], improve self-efficacy levels of patients with heart failure [65], and have a positive effect on some diabetes-related cardiovascular risk factors (e.g., glycemic control) [66], among others. These findings, along with our results, suggest that internal HLC has a significant impact on factors related to HRQoL that are relevant to CVD patients. This highlights the need to prioritize psychological treatments that promote and enhance this construct, which may prove effective in improving HRQoL and reducing cardiovascular risk factors.

On the other hand, a negative prediction of other people HLC was found over HRQoL. These findings are consistent with previous studies [61,67]. Blaming external factors for one's health may lead to a perception of a lack of control and autonomy in the health–disease process. In the context of cardiac care, this may negatively impact CVD patients' self-efficacy, leading to poor adherence to medication and other essential healthy behaviors, such as a healthy diet and physical activity, which are crucial for effective disease management and a good quality of life [68–71]. These results support the need to consider the influence of external HLC when implementing policies and interventions aimed at promoting healthy behaviors of these patients [72]. Therefore, the findings of this study underscore the importance of promoting patient empowerment, autonomy, and patient responsibility in healthcare interventions in order to mitigate the lack of perceived control over their own health that may affect the quality of life of these patients.

4.1. Practical Implications

This longitudinal study has allowed us to test the predictive hypotheses proposed supporting the potential relevance of a clinical intervention based on providing patients with a positive approach and strengthening their internal locus of control. In line with previous literature that has reported a well-known relationship between psychological variables and CVD risk factors and CVH [6,9], the present findings provide evidence of the role of these psychological variables in the quality of life and anxiety and depressive symptoms in chronic patients [73,74]. Positivity and HLC may also influence the management of CVD, given their association with other psychological variables that are key to a better understanding and management of the disease [11,18,39], such as self-efficacy [65]. This association may, hence, promote CVH (e.g., healthier diet, better adherence to treatment, and quitting smoking) with significant positive outcomes among these patients [68]. Therefore, healthcare providers may incorporate strategies that focus on building positivity and self-perception of control as part of a comprehensive treatment plan for CVD patients to improve their overall health and well-being. Accordingly, the results of this study add interesting information to be considered in future CVD interventions such as cardiac rehabilitation programs, as well as emerging healthcare trends, such as tailored interventions [75] or telemedicine [76].

4.2. Limitations and Future Research

There are some limitations in this study that need to be acknowledged and considered for future research. Firstly, the use of self-reporting questionnaires, even with validated instruments and guaranteed confidentiality and anonymity, can introduce bias into the data by relying solely on subjective reporting. Future studies may incorporate a multi-method assessment in order to obtain more accurate information and reduce social desirability when collecting data (e.g., including external validation, honesty scales, etc.). In addition, the magnitude of the reported correlations could be considered as weak and/or moderate according to Cohen (1988) [56]. However, recent literature criticizes the use of Cohen's cut-off and proposes a more flexible classification [77], which would give our results greater power and validity. In any case, given the potential relevance of these results for therapeutic interventions, future studies with larger samples would be needed to detect stronger relationships between these variables. In line with this, to obtain a better understanding of the trajectory of outcomes and increase the statistical power, future studies may benefit from including more follow-up evaluations. The underrepresentation of women in this study sample may hinder the generalizability of the findings to the female population with CVD. Additionally, the possible influence of other variables has not been studied (for example, a stressful event between assessments). Given the demonstrated relevance of anxiety, depression, and HRQoL in chronic and CVD patients, it is utterly important to conduct further research in this area to explore and study the variables that impact patients' psychological well-being and to measure the disease prognosis associated with psychological states. This would enable the development of new psychological interventions that consider the influence of these variables, aiming to enhance the well-being of these patients and improve their quality of life.

5. Conclusions

This study highlights the important role that positivity and HLC play in psychological health outcomes for CVD patients. These findings suggest that promoting a positive orientation and internal HLC may lead to improved psychological well-being, reduced anxiety and depression levels, and enhanced HRQoL among these patients. In conclusion, this study's results underline the importance of considering patients' psychological well-being in the context of cardiac rehabilitation, and suggest that interventions focused on a psychological approach may be beneficial for enhancing CVH and a better prognosis for these patients. Further studies are required in this direction in order to empirically investigate the effectiveness of incorporating this approach in cardiac care.

Author Contributions: Conceptualization, C.T., B.L. and R.C.-M.; methodology, C.T., B.L. and R.C.-M.; software, B.L. and R.C.-M.; validation, C.T., B.L., R.C.-M., N.Z.F.-M., E.C. and M.V.; formal analysis, R.C.-M. and N.Z.F.-M.; investigation, C.T., B.L., R.C.-M., N.Z.F.-M., E.C. and M.V.; resources, B.L. and C.T.; data curation, R.C.-M. and M.V.; writing—original draft preparation, B.L., R.C.-M. and N.Z.F.-M.; writing—review and editing, C.T. and N.Z.F.-M.; visualization, C.T., B.L., R.C.-M. and N.Z.F.-M.; supervision, C.T., B.L. and R.C.-M.; project administration, C.T. and B.L.; funding acquisition, C.T. and B.L. All authors have read and agreed to the published version of the manuscript.

Funding: This research received no external funding.

Institutional Review Board Statement: This study was conducted in accordance with the Declaration of Helsinki. The Institutional Review Board Statement is not applicable considering the retrospective nature of the study.

Informed Consent Statement: Informed consent has been obtained from the patient(s) to publish this paper, if applicable.

Data Availability Statement: The data presented in this study are available on request from the corresponding author.

Conflicts of Interest: The authors declare no conflict of interest.

References

1. Cardiovascular Disease. Available online: https://www.nhs.uk/conditions/cardiovascular-disease/ (accessed on 20 April 2023).
2. Roth, G.A.; Mensah, G.A.; Johnson, C.O.; Addolorato, G.; Ammirati, E.; Baddour, L.M.; Barengo, N.C.; Beaton, A.Z.; Benjamin, E.J.; Benziger, C.P.; et al. Global Burden of Cardiovascular Diseases and Risk Factors, 1990–2019. *J. Am. Coll. Cardiol.* **2020**, *76*, 2982–3021. [CrossRef] [PubMed]
3. The Top 10 Causes of Death. Available online: https://www.who.int/news-room/fact-sheets/detail/the-top-10-causes-of-death (accessed on 31 March 2023).
4. Non Communicable Diseases. Available online: https://www.who.int/news-room/fact-sheets/detail/noncommunicable-diseases (accessed on 20 April 2023).

5. Townsend, N.; Kazakiewicz, D.; Lucy Wright, F.; Timmis, A.; Huculeci, R.; Torbica, A.; Gale, C.P.; Achenbach, S.; Weidinger, F.; Vardas, P. Epidemiology of Cardiovascular Disease in Europe. *Nat. Rev. Cardiol.* **2022**, *19*, 133–143. [CrossRef] [PubMed]
6. Levine, G.N.; Cohen, B.E.; Commodore-Mensah, Y.; Fleury, J.; Huffman, J.C.; Khalid, U.; Labarthe, D.R.; Lavretsky, H.; Michos, E.D.; Spatz, E.S.; et al. Psychological Health, Well-Being, and the Mind-Heart-Body Connection: A Scientific Statement From the American Heart Association. *Circulation* **2021**, *143*, e763–e783. [CrossRef] [PubMed]
7. Pedersen, S.S.; Andersen, C.M. Minding the Heart: Why Are We Still Not Closer to Treating Depression and Anxiety in Clinical Cardiology Practice? *Eur. J. Prev. Cardiol.* **2018**, *25*, 244–246. [CrossRef]
8. Helmark, C.; Harrison, A.; Pedersen, S.S.; Doherty, P. Systematic Screening for Anxiety and Depression in Cardiac Rehabilitation—Are We There Yet? *Int. J. Cardiol.* **2022**, *352*, 65–71. [CrossRef]
9. Pogosova, N.; Saner, H.; Pedersen, S.S.; Cupples, M.E.; McGee, H.; Höfer, S.; Doyle, F.; Schmid, J.-P.; von Känel, R.; Cardiac Rehabilitation Section of the European Association of Cardiovascular Prevention and Rehabilitation of the European Society of Cardiology. Psychosocial Aspects in Cardiac Rehabilitation: From Theory to Practice. A Position Paper from the Cardiac Rehabilitation Section of the European Association of Cardiovascular Prevention and Rehabilitation of the European Society of Cardiology. *Eur. J. Prev. Cardiol.* **2015**, *22*, 1290–1306. [CrossRef]
10. Visseren, F.L.J.; Mach, F.; Smulders, Y.M.; Carballo, D.; Koskinas, K.C.; Bäck, M.; Benetos, A.; Biffi, A.; Boavida, J.-M.; Capodanno, D.; et al. 2021 ESC Guidelines on Cardiovascular Disease Prevention in Clinical Practice: Developed by the Task Force for Cardiovascular Disease Prevention in Clinical Practice with Representatives of the European Society of Cardiology and 12 Medical Societies With the Special Contribution of the European Association of Preventive Cardiology (EAPC). *Eur. Heart J.* **2021**, *42*, 3227–3337. [CrossRef]
11. Kubzansky, L.D.; Huffman, J.C.; Boehm, J.K.; Hernandez, R.; Kim, E.S.; Koga, H.K.; Feig, E.H.; Lloyd-Jones, D.M.; Seligman, M.E.P.; Labarthe, D.R. Positive Psychological Well-Being and Cardiovascular Disease: JACC Health Promotion Series. *J. Am. Coll. Cardiol.* **2018**, *72*, 1382–1396. [CrossRef]
12. Bosworth, H.B.; Blalock, D.V.; Hoyle, R.H.; Czajkowski, S.M.; Voils, C.I. The Role of Psychological Science in Efforts to Improve Cardiovascular Medication Adherence. *Am. Psychol.* **2018**, *73*, 968–980. [CrossRef]
13. Pedersen, S.S.; von Känel, R.; Tully, P.J.; Denollet, J. Psychosocial Perspectives in Cardiovascular Disease. *Eur. J. Prev. Cardiol.* **2017**, *24*, 108–115. [CrossRef]
14. Pedersen, S.S.; Doyle, F. Effectiveness of Psychological Intervention as Add-on to Standard Cardiac Rehabilitation: Time to Adopt New Methods or Keep Doing More of the Same? *Eur. J. Prev. Cardiol.* **2019**, *26*, 1032–1034. [CrossRef] [PubMed]
15. Ryff, C.D. Happiness Is Everything, or Is It? Explorations on the Meaning of Psychological Well-Being. *J. Personal. Soc. Psychol.* **1989**, *57*, 1069–1081. [CrossRef]
16. Kobasa, S.C. Stressful Life Events, Personality, and Health: An Inquiry into Hardiness. *J. Personal. Soc. Psychol.* **1979**, *37*, 1–11. [CrossRef] [PubMed]
17. Massé, R.; Poulin, C.; Dassa, C.; Lambert, J.; Bélair, S.; Battaglini, A. The Structure of Mental Health: Higher-Order Confirmatory Factor Analyses of Psychological Distress and Well-Being Measures. *Soc. Indic. Res.* **1998**, *45*, 475–504. [CrossRef]
18. Luque, B.; García, M.d.M.R.; Cuadrado, E.; Gutiérrez, T.; Castillo, R.; Arenas, A.; Tabernero, C. Comparative Study of Positivity and Self-Efficacy for the Regulation of Negative Emotions in Persons with and without Cardiovascular Disease. *EC Psychol. Psychiatr* **2017**, *4*, 247–263.
19. Farhane-Medina, N.Z.; Castillo-Mayén, R.; Luque, B.; Rubio, S.J.; Gutiérrez-Domingo, T.; Cuadrado, E.; Arenas, A.; Tabernero, C. A Brief MHealth-Based Psychological Intervention in Emotion Regulation to Promote Positive Subjective Well-Being in Cardiovascular Disease Patients: A Non-Randomized Controlled Trial. *Healthcare* **2022**, *10*, 1640. [CrossRef] [PubMed]
20. Boehm, J.K.; Soo, J.; Chen, Y.; Zevon, E.S.; Hernandez, R.; Lloyd-Jones, D.; Kubzansky, L.D. Psychological Well-Being's Link with Cardiovascular Health in Older Adults. *Am. J. Prev. Med.* **2017**, *53*, 791–798. [CrossRef]
21. Ogunmoroti, O.; Osibogun, O.; Spatz, E.S.; Okunrintemi, V.; Mathews, L.; Ndumele, C.E.; Michos, E.D. A Systematic Review of the Bidirectional Relationship between Depressive Symptoms and Cardiovascular Health. *Prev. Med.* **2022**, *154*, 106891. [CrossRef]
22. Gan, Y.; Gong, Y.; Tong, X.; Sun, H.; Cong, Y.; Dong, X.; Wang, Y.; Xu, X.; Yin, X.; Deng, J.; et al. Depression and the Risk of Coronary Heart Disease: A Meta-Analysis of Prospective Cohort Studies. *BMC Psychiatry* **2014**, *14*, 371. [CrossRef]
23. Cohen, B.E.; Edmondson, D.; Kronish, I.M. State of the Art Review: Depression, Stress, Anxiety, and Cardiovascular Disease. *Am. J. Hypertens.* **2015**, *28*, 1295–1302. [CrossRef]
24. Batelaan, N.M.; Seldenrijk, A.; Bot, M.; van Balkom, A.J.L.M.; Penninx, B.W.J.H. Anxiety and New Onset of Cardiovascular Disease: Critical Review and Meta-Analysis. *Br. J. Psychiatry* **2016**, *208*, 223–231. [CrossRef] [PubMed]
25. Rawashdeh, S.I.; Ibdah, R.; Kheirallah, K.A.; Al-Kasasbeh, A.; Raffee, L.A.; Alrabadi, N.; Albustami, I.S.; Haddad, R.; Ibdah, R.M.; Al-Mistarehi, A.-H. Prevalence Estimates, Severity, and Risk Factors of Depressive Symptoms among Coronary Artery Disease Patients after Ten Days of Percutaneous Coronary Intervention. *Clin. Pract. Epidemiol. Ment. Health* **2021**, *17*, 103–113. [CrossRef] [PubMed]
26. Gathright, E.C.; Goldstein, C.M.; Josephson, R.A.; Hughes, J.W. Depression Increases the Risk of Mortality in Patients with Heart Failure: A Meta-Analysis. *J. Psychosom. Res.* **2017**, *94*, 82–89. [CrossRef] [PubMed]
27. Allabadi, H.; Probst-Hensch, N.; Alkaiyat, A.; Haj-Yahia, S.; Schindler, C.; Kwiatkowski, M.; Zemp, E. Mediators of Gender Effects on Depression among Cardiovascular Disease Patients in Palestine. *BMC Psychiatry* **2019**, *19*, 284. [CrossRef]

28. Serpytis, P.; Navickas, P.; Lukaviciute, L.; Navickas, A.; Aranauskas, R.; Serpytis, R.; Deksnyte, A.; Glaveckaite, S.; Petrulioniene, Z.; Samalavicius, R. Gender-Based Differences in Anxiety and Depression Following Acute Myocardial Infarction. *Arq. Bras. Cardiol.* 2018, *111*, 676–683. [CrossRef]
29. Conley, S.; Feder, S.; Redeker, N.S. The Relationship between Pain, Fatigue, Depression and Functional Performance in Stable Heart Failure. *Heart Lung* 2015, *44*, 107–112. [CrossRef]
30. Ko, H.-Y.; Lee, J.-K.; Shin, J.-Y.; Jo, E. Health-Related Quality of Life and Cardiovascular Disease Risk in Korean Adults. *Korean J. Fam. Med.* 2015, *36*, 349–356. [CrossRef]
31. Rieckmann, N.; Neumann, K.; Feger, S.; Ibes, P.; Napp, A.; Preuß, D.; Dreger, H.; Feuchtner, G.; Plank, F.; Suchánek, V.; et al. Health-Related Qualify of Life, Angina Type and Coronary Artery Disease in Patients with Stable Chest Pain. *Health Qual. Life Outcomes* 2020, *18*, 140. [CrossRef]
32. Yin, S.; Njai, R.; Barker, L.; Siegel, P.Z.; Liao, Y. Summarizing Health-Related Quality of Life (HRQOL): Development and Testing of a One-Factor Model. *Popul. Health Metr.* 2016, *14*, 22. [CrossRef]
33. Al-Noumani, H.; Al Omari, O.; Al-Naamani, Z. Role of Health Literacy, Social Support, Patient-Physician Relationship, and Health-Related Quality of Life in Predicting Medication Adherence in Cardiovascular Diseases in Oman. *Patient Prefer. Adherence* 2023, *17*, 643–652. [CrossRef]
34. Pinheiro, L.C.; Reshetnyak, E.; Sterling, M.R.; Richman, J.S.; Kern, L.M.; Safford, M.M. Using Health-Related Quality of Life to Predict Cardiovascular Disease Events. *Qual. Life Res.* 2019, *28*, 1465–1475. [CrossRef] [PubMed]
35. Phyo, A.Z.Z.; Ryan, J.; Gonzalez-Chica, D.A.; Stocks, N.P.; Reid, C.M.; Tonkin, A.M.; Woods, R.L.; Nelson, M.R.; Murray, A.M.; Gasevic, D.; et al. Health-Related Quality of Life and Incident Cardiovascular Disease Events in Community-Dwelling Older People: A Prospective Cohort Study. *Int. J. Cardiol.* 2021, *339*, 170–178. [CrossRef] [PubMed]
36. Ryckman, R.M. *Theories of Personality*, 8th ed.; Wadsworth/Thomson Learning: Belmont, CA, USA, 2004; pp. xxii, 698, ISBN 978-0-534-61983-1.
37. Caprara, G.V.; Alessandri, G.; Eisenberg, N.; Kupfer, A.; Steca, P.; Caprara, M.G.; Yamaguchi, S.; Fukuzawa, A.; Abela, J. The Positivity Scale. *Psychol. Assess.* 2012, *24*, 701–712. [CrossRef] [PubMed]
38. Qin, Z.; Mei, S.; Gao, T.; Liang, L.; Li, C.; Hu, Y.; Guo, X.; Meng, C.; Lv, J.; Yuan, T.; et al. Self-Esteem as a Mediator between Life Satisfaction and Depression among Cardiovascular Disease Patients. *Clin. Nurs. Res.* 2022, *31*, 115–121. [CrossRef] [PubMed]
39. Amonoo, H.L.; Celano, C.M.; Sadlonova, M.; Huffman, J.C. Is Optimism a Protective Factor for Cardiovascular Disease? *Curr. Cardiol. Rep.* 2021, *23*, 158. [CrossRef]
40. Boehm, J.K.; Kubzansky, L.D. The Heart's Content: The Association between Positive Psychological Well-Being and Cardiovascular Health. *Psychol. Bull.* 2012, *138*, 655–691. [CrossRef]
41. DuBois, C.M.; Lopez, O.V.; Beale, E.E.; Healy, B.C.; Boehm, J.K.; Huffman, J.C. Relationships between Positive Psychological Constructs and Health Outcomes in Patients with Cardiovascular Disease: A Systematic Review. *Int. J. Cardiol.* 2015, *195*, 265–280. [CrossRef]
42. Araújo-Soares, V.; Hankonen, N.; Presseau, J.; Rodrigues, A.; Sniehotta, F.F. Developing Behavior Change Interventions for Self-Management in Chronic Illness. *Eur. Psychol.* 2019, *24*, 7–25. [CrossRef]
43. Wallston, B.S.; Wallston, K.A.; Kaplan, G.D.; Maides, S.A. Development and Validation of the Health Locus of Control (HLC) Scale. *J. Consult. Clin. Psychol.* 1976, *44*, 580–585. [CrossRef]
44. Waller, K.V.; Bates, R.C. Health Locus of Control and Self-Efficacy Beliefs in a Healthy Elderly Sample. *Am. J. Health Promot.* 1992, *6*, 302–309. [CrossRef]
45. Pharr, J.; Enejoh, V.; Mavegam, B.O.; Olutola, A.; Karick, H.; Ezeanolue, E.E. Relationship between Health Locus of Control and Risky Sexual Behaviors among Nigerian Adolescents. *J. AIDS Clin. Res.* 2015, *6*, 471. [CrossRef] [PubMed]
46. Wallston, K.A.; Wallston, B.S.; DeVellis, R. Development of the Multidimensional Health Locus of Control (MHLC) Scales. *Health Educ. Monogr.* 1978, *6*, 160–170. [CrossRef] [PubMed]
47. Berglund, E.; Lytsy, P.; Westerling, R. The Influence of Locus of Control on Self-Rated Health in Context of Chronic Disease: A Structural Equation Modeling Approach in a Cross Sectional Study. *BMC Public Health* 2014, *14*, 492. [CrossRef] [PubMed]
48. Delgado-Lista, J.; Perez-Martinez, P.; Garcia-Rios, A.; Alcala-Diaz, J.F.; Perez-Caballero, A.I.; Gomez-Delgado, F.; Fuentes, F.; Quintana-Navarro, G.; Lopez-Segura, F.; Ortiz-Morales, A.M.; et al. CORonary Diet Intervention with Olive Oil and Cardiovascular PREVention Study (the CORDIOPREV Study): Rationale, Methods, and Baseline Characteristics: A Clinical Trial Comparing the Efficacy of a Mediterranean Diet Rich in Olive Oil versus a Low-Fat Diet on Cardiovascular Disease in Coronary Patients. *Am. Heart J.* 2016, *177*, 42–50. [CrossRef] [PubMed]
49. Delgado-Lista, J.; Alcala-Diaz, J.F.; Torres-Peña, J.D.; Quintana-Navarro, G.M.; Fuentes, F.; Garcia-Rios, A.; Ortiz-Morales, A.M.; Gonzalez-Requero, A.I.; Perez-Caballero, A.I.; Yubero-Serrano, E.M.; et al. Long-Term Secondary Prevention of Cardiovascular Disease with a Mediterranean Diet and a Low-Fat Diet (CORDIOPREV): A Randomised Controlled Trial. *Lancet* 2022, *399*, 1876–1885. [CrossRef]
50. Zigmond, A.S.; Snaith, R.P. The Hospital Anxiety and Depression Scale. *Acta Psychiatr. Scand.* 1983, *67*, 361–370. [CrossRef]
51. Terol, M.C.; López-Roig, S.; Rodríguez-Marín, J.; Martín-Aragón, M.; Pastor, M.A.; Reig, M.T. Propiedades Psicométricas de La Escala Hospitalaria de Ansiedad y Depresión (HAD) En Población Española. [Hospital Anxiety and Depression Scale (HAD): Psychometric Properties in Spanish Population.]. *Ansiedad Estrés* 2007, *13*, 163–176.
52. Ware, J.; Kosinski, M.; Keller, S.D. A 12-Item Short-Form Health Survey: Construction of Scales and Preliminary Tests of Reliability and Validity. *Med. Care* 1996, *34*, 220–233. [CrossRef]

53. Failde, I.; Medina, P.; Ramirez, C.; Arana, R. Construct and Criterion Validity of the SF-12 Health Questionnaire in Patients with Acute Myocardial Infarction and Unstable Angina. *J. Eval. Clin. Pract.* **2010**, *16*, 569–573. [CrossRef]
54. Vilagut, G.; Valderas, J.M.; Ferrer, M.; Garin, O.; López-García, E.; Alonso, J. [Interpretation of SF-36 and SF-12 questionnaires in Spain: Physical and mental components]. *Med. Clin.* **2008**, *130*, 726–735. [CrossRef]
55. Schermelleh-Engel, K.; Moosbrugger, H.; Müller, H. Evaluating the Fit of Structural Equation Models: Tests of Significance and Descriptive Goodness-of-Fit Measures. *Methods Psychol. Res.* **2003**, *8*, 23–74.
56. Cohen, J. *Statistical Power Analysis for the Behavioral Sciences*, 2nd ed.; Routledge: New York, NY, USA, 1988; ISBN 978-0-203-77158-7.
57. Alessandri, G.; Caprara, G.V.; Tisak, J. The Unique Contribution of Positive Orientation to Optimal Functioning: Further Explorations. *Eur. Psychol.* **2012**, *17*, 44–54. [CrossRef]
58. Sahoo, S.; Padhy, S.K.; Padhee, B.; Singla, N.; Sarkar, S. Role of Personality in Cardiovascular Diseases: An Issue That Needs to Be Focused Too! *Indian Heart J.* **2018**, *70* (Suppl. 3), S471–S477. [CrossRef]
59. Steca, P.; Monzani, D.; Pierobon, A.; Avvenuti, G.; Greco, A.; Giardini, A. Measuring Dispositional Optimism in Patients with Chronic Heart Failure and Their Healthcare Providers: The Validity of the Life Orientation Test-Revised. *Patient Prefer. Adherence* **2017**, *11*, 1497–1503. [CrossRef] [PubMed]
60. Caprara, G.V.; Eisenberg, N.; Alessandri, G. Positivity: The Dispositional Basis of Happiness. *J. Happiness Stud.* **2017**, *18*, 353–371. [CrossRef]
61. Mercer, D.A.; Ditto, B.; Lavoie, K.L.; Campbell, T.; Arsenault, A.; Bacon, S.L. Health Locus of Control Is Associated With Physical Activity and Other Health Behaviors in Cardiac Patients. *J. Cardiopulm. Rehabil. Prev.* **2018**, *38*, 394–399. [CrossRef]
62. Lindström, M.; Rosvall, M. Health Locus of Control and Mortality: A Population-Based Prospective Cohort Study. *Public Health* **2020**, *185*, 209–211. [CrossRef]
63. Milte, C.M.; Luszcz, M.A.; Ratcliffe, J.; Masters, S.; Crotty, M. Influence of Health Locus of Control on Recovery of Function in Recently Hospitalized Frail Older Adults. *Geriatr. Gerontol. Int.* **2015**, *15*, 341–349. [CrossRef]
64. Musich, S.; Wang, S.S.; Slindee, L.; Kraemer, S.; Yeh, C.S. The Impact of Internal Locus of Control on Healthcare Utilization, Expenditures, and Health Status across Older Adult Income Levels. *Geriatr. Nurs.* **2020**, *41*, 274–281. [CrossRef]
65. Moradi, Y.; Shara, S.A.A.; Namadi, F.; Mollazadeh, F. The Relationship between Health Locus of Control and Self-Efficacy in Patients with Heart Failure. *Nurs. Midwifery Stud.* **2022**, *11*, 31. [CrossRef]
66. Williams, J.S.; Lynch, C.P.; Voronca, D.; Egede, L.E. Health Locus of Control and Cardiovascular Risk Factors in Veterans with Type 2 Diabetes. *Endocrine* **2016**, *51*, 83–90. [CrossRef]
67. Rizza, F.; Gison, A.; Bonassi, S.; Dall'Armi, V.; Tonto, F.; Giaquinto, S. "Locus of Control", Health-Related Quality of Life, Emotional Distress and Disability in Parkinson's Disease. *J. Health Psychol.* **2017**, *22*, 844–852. [CrossRef] [PubMed]
68. Banik, A.; Schwarzer, R.; Knoll, N.; Czekierda, K.; Luszczynska, A. Self-Efficacy and Quality of Life among People with Cardiovascular Diseases: A Meta-Analysis. *Rehabil. Psychol.* **2018**, *63*, 295–312. [CrossRef] [PubMed]
69. Pakaya, R.E.; Syam, Y.; Syahrul, S. Correlation of Self-Efficacy and Self-Care of Patients Undergoing Hemodialysis with Their Quality of Life. *Enfermería Clínica* **2021**, *31*, S797–S801. [CrossRef]
70. Nguyen, T.T.N.; Liang, S.-Y.; Liu, C.-Y.; Chien, C.-H. Self-Care Self-Efficacy and Depression Associated with Quality of Life among Patients Undergoing Hemodialysis in Vietnam. *PLoS ONE* **2022**, *17*, e0270100. [CrossRef]
71. Wang, R.; Zhou, C.; Wu, Y.; Sun, M.; Yang, L.; Ye, X.; Zhang, M. Patient Empowerment and Self-Management Behaviour of Chronic Disease Patients: A Moderated Mediation Model of Self-Efficacy and Health Locus of Control. *J. Adv. Nurs.* **2022**, *78*, 1055–1065. [CrossRef] [PubMed]
72. Grisolía, J.M.; Longo, A.; Hutchinson, G.; Kee, F. Applying Health Locus of Control and Latent Class Modelling to Food and Physical Activity Choices Affecting CVD Risk. *Soc. Sci. Med.* **2015**, *132*, 1–10. [CrossRef]
73. Caprara, G.V.; Castellani, V.; Alessandri, G.; Mazzuca, F.; La Torre, M.; Barbaranelli, C.; Colaiaco, F.; Gerbino, M.; Pasquali, V.; D'Amelio, R.; et al. Being Positive despite Illness: The Contribution of Positivity to the Quality of Life of Cancer Patients. *Psychol. Health* **2016**, *31*, 524–534. [CrossRef]
74. Tabernero, C.; Caprara, G.V.; Gutiérrez-Domingo, T.; Cuadrado, E.; Castillo-Mayén, R.; Arenas, A.; Rubio, S.; Luque, B. Positivity and Self-Efficacy Beliefs Explaining Health-Related Quality of Life in Cardiovascular Patients. *Psicothema* **2021**, *33*, 433–441. [CrossRef]
75. Xu, H.-Y.; Yu, Y.-J.; Zhang, Q.-H.; Hu, H.-Y.; Li, M. Tailored Interventions to Improve Medication Adherence for Cardiovascular Diseases. *Front. Pharmacol.* **2020**, *11*, 510339. [CrossRef]
76. Cruz-Ramos, N.A.; Alor-Hernández, G.; Colombo-Mendoza, L.O.; Sánchez-Cervantes, J.L.; Rodríguez-Mazahua, L.; Guarneros-Nolasco, L.R. MHealth Apps for Self-Management of Cardiovascular Diseases: A Scoping Review. *Healthcare* **2022**, *10*, 322. [CrossRef] [PubMed]
77. Gignac, G.E.; Szodorai, E.T. Effect Size Guidelines for Individual Differences Researchers. *Personal. Individ. Differ.* **2016**, *102*, 74–78. [CrossRef]

Disclaimer/Publisher's Note: The statements, opinions and data contained in all publications are solely those of the individual author(s) and contributor(s) and not of MDPI and/or the editor(s). MDPI and/or the editor(s) disclaim responsibility for any injury to people or property resulting from any ideas, methods, instructions or products referred to in the content.

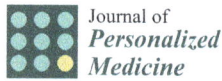

Article

Stroke Risk in Young Women with Primary Dysmenorrhea: A Propensity-Score-Matched Retrospective Cohort Study

Chung-Hsin Yeh [1,2], Fung-Chang Sung [3,4,5,*,†], Chih-Hsin Muo [3], Pao-Sheng Yen [6,*,†] and Chung Y. Hsu [3,7]

1. Department of Nursing, College of Nursing and Health Sciences, Da-Yeh University, Changhua 515, Taiwan
2. Department of Neurology, Yuan Rung Hospital, Changhua 510, Taiwan
3. Management Office for Health Data, China Medical University Hospital, Taichung 404, Taiwan
4. Department of Health Services Administration, China Medical University College of Public Health, Taichung 406, Taiwan
5. Department of Food Nutrition and Health Biotechnology, Asia University, Taichung 413, Taiwan
6. Department of Neuroradiology, Kuang Tien General Hospital, Taichung 433, Taiwan
7. Graduate Institute of Biomedical Sciences, China Medical University, Taichung 404, Taiwan
* Correspondence: fcsung1008@yahoo.com (F.-C.S.); bert.yen@gmail.com (P.-S.Y.)
† These authors contributed equally to this work.

Abstract: Background: Studies on strokes associated with dysmenorrhea are limited. We conducted a propensity-score-matched retrospective cohort study to assess the risk of stroke in women with primary dysmenorrhea (PD). Methods: From the claims data of one million people in Taiwan's insurance program, we identified 18,783 women aged 15–40 years, newly diagnosed with PD in 2000–2010, without a history of stroke. We randomly selected a comparison cohort without stroke history and dysmenorrhea, with the same sample size matched by age, index date, and propensity score. We began a follow-up with individuals one year after cohort entry to the end of 2013 to capture stroke events. Results: The two study cohorts were well-matched for age and comorbidities, with 54% of women aged 15–24. Stroke incidence was 1.5-fold higher in the PD cohort than in the comparison cohort (6.05 vs. 4.01 per 10,000 person-years, or 99 vs. 65 cases), with an adjusted hazard ratio (aHR) of 1.51 (95%CI 1.11–2.06) after adjustment for matched pairs. Nearly 70% of strokes were ischemic strokes, which occurred 1.6 times more frequently in the PD cohort than in the comparison cohort (4.40 vs. 2.71 per 10,000 person-years, or 72 vs. 44 cases), aHR = 1.61 (95% CI 1.11–2.33), after adjustment for matched pairs. The incidence of hemorrhagic stroke was also higher in the PD cohort than in the comparison cohort (1.65 vs. 1.29 per 10,000 person-years, or 27 versus 21 cases), but the difference was not significant. Conclusion: Women of reproductive age with PD are at increased risk for ischemic stroke.

Keywords: dysmenorrhea; propensity score; retrospective cohort study; stroke

Citation: Yeh, C.-H.; Sung, F.-C.; Muo, C.-H.; Yen, P.-S.; Hsu, C.Y. Stroke Risk in Young Women with Primary Dysmenorrhea: A Propensity-Score-Matched Retrospective Cohort Study. *J. Pers. Med.* **2023**, *13*, 114. https://doi.org/10.3390/jpm13010114

Academic Editor: Georgios Samanidis

Received: 15 October 2022
Revised: 26 December 2022
Accepted: 30 December 2022
Published: 4 January 2023

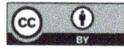

Copyright: © 2023 by the authors. Licensee MDPI, Basel, Switzerland. This article is an open access article distributed under the terms and conditions of the Creative Commons Attribution (CC BY) license (https://creativecommons.org/licenses/by/4.0/).

1. Introduction

Women go through a menstrual cycle due to the monthly change in estrogen production. The menstruation period begins with menarche and ends after menopause. Dysmenorrhea is a painful condition for women during menstruation in which they experience an intense sensation of pain or even cramping in the lower abdomen. Adolescents and young women with severe and frequent cramps and pain from dysmenorrhea tend to be regularly absent from school and work [1,2]. Absence from daily work during the dysmenorrhea cycle may be responsible for the loss of 600 million work hours in the United States [3].

A previous review of the international literature of 178 studies found that the prevalence of dysmenorrhea varied widely by ethnic group, ranging from 16.8% to 81% [4]. The age of women is inversely related to the prevalence, which is higher in young women aged 17–24 years, and more than half suffer from the condition [5,6]. There are two types of dysmenorrhea. Primary dysmenorrhea (PD) presents with lower abdominal pain without evident organic pelvic disease and is more common in younger women after their menstrual cycle is established. Secondary dysmenorrhea (SD) is associated with disorders of the reproductive organs [5,7]. The prevalence of PD in women may be up to six times higher than those with SD [8]. These disorders also vary in Asian women. It has been estimated that 15.8–78.5% of Japanese women suffer from PD [9,10], with more than 60% having moderate to severe lower abdominal cramps [10] and almost half resorting to self-medication [9]. Prevalence rates in Taiwan and Korea were 70.7% and 75.1%, respectively [11–13], higher than those reported for women in China, ranging from 41.7 to 56.4% [2,14]. A cross-sectional study in secondary schools in Kuala Lumpur, Malaysia, reported that 79.7% of Malaysian girls, 69.8% of Chinese girls, and 82.4% of Indian girls had suffered from dysmenorrhea [15]. Dysmenorrhea symptoms might differ between White and Asian women. White women generally experience more intense and longer-lasting pain [16].

Stroke is the third leading cause of death globally and one of main causes of disability [17]. Approximately 15 million new stroke patients are diagnosed annually worldwide [18]. With one stroke event every 40 s, it is also the third leading cause of death among women in the United States [19,20]. The Framingham Heart Study found that strokes occur less frequently in women than men in the younger population [21]. Female stroke patients tend to present worse sequelae than male stroke patients [22,23]. A case–control study examining Taiwanese women with dysmenorrhea aged 15–49 years found an increased risk of stroke with age, significant for those aged 30 years and older [24]. Hypertension is also a significant risk factor for stroke, with an adjusted odds ratio of 4.53. However, types of dysmenorrhea were not addressed in these studies.

The complicated pathophysiology of PD is associated with the overexpression of prostaglandin. Prostaglandin is thought to be one of the mediators of chronic vascular inflammation, which has been linked to heart disease and stroke [3,25]. A recent study found that women with PD have an increased risk of ischemic heart disease [26]. Women with PD may also be at higher risk for stroke. To our knowledge, no study has investigated stroke risk specifically for women with PD. Because PD is more prevalent in women than SD, we conducted a study to examine the risk of stroke in women with PD using insurance claims data from Taiwan.

2. Methods
2.1. Data Source

In this retrospective cohort study, we used the Longitudinal Health Insurance Database (LHID) with claims data of one million insured persons randomly selected from the National Health Insurance Research Database (NHIRD) established by the National Health Insurance Administration of Taiwan. The insurance system was established in 1995 as a mandatory enrollment program, with over 99% of Taiwan's 23.72 million residents covered. The database contains medical records of outpatients and inpatients and demographic data from 1996 to 2013. Diseases are coded using the International Classification of Diseases, Ninth Revision, Clinical Modification (ICD 9-CM), and the Anatomical Therapeutic Chemical (ATC) classification system. In addition, all identification numbers of insured persons in the claims data were re-coded before being made available to users to protect privacy. This study was approved by the Research Ethics Committee of China Medical University and Hospital in Taiwan (CMUH104-REC2-115 (CR-4)).

2.2. Study Population

From LHID claims data, we identified 35,977 women with dysmenorrhea (ICD-9-CM 625.3) newly diagnosed between 2000 and 2010 with at least two consecutive diagnoses as the potential study population. The date of the first dysmenorrhea diagnosis was defined as the index date. Patients with only one diagnosis were not selected to avoid coding and/or medical billing errors. To create the study cohorts, women aged <15 or >40 years with a history of stroke, endometriosis, uterine myoma or pelvic inflammatory disease, hysterectomy, ovariectomy, or cancer, or aspirin use were excluded (Figure 1). We also excluded women with follow-up duration <1 year due to death, stroke, or withdrawal from the insurance. Women aged 41–49 years old were also excluded to avoid the potential impact of premenopausal and early menopause. Excluding women with diagnoses of obvious gynecologic conditions resulted in the exclusion of women with SD [27,28]. The same exclusion criteria were applied to women without dysmenorrhea for comparisons. From the remaining 18,812 women with dysmenorrhea and 101,154 women without dysmenorrhea, we established a PD cohort and a comparison cohort matched by age, index date, and propensity score. We randomly assigned an index date for each comparison woman. We estimated the propensity score for each woman using logistic regression to estimate the probability of disease status on the basis of the baseline variables of age; index date; and comorbidities including diabetes (ICD-9 code: 250; A code: A181), hypertension (ICD-9 code: 401–405; A codes: A260 and A269), hyperlipidemia (ICD-9 codes: 272.0, 272.1, 272.2, 272.3, and 272.4), obesity (ICD-9 codes: 278, A183), alcoholism (ICD-9 codes: 291, 303, 305.00, 305.01, 305.02, 305.03, 790.3, and V11.3), arrhythmia (ICD-9 code: 427), thyroid disease (ICD-9 code: 240–246), migraine (ICD-9 code: 346), immune disorders (ICD-9 code: 279), systemic lupus erythematosus (ICD-9 code: 710.0), and rheumatoid arthritis (ICD-9 code: 714.0). All comorbidities were defined before the index date, with at least two consecutive diagnoses.

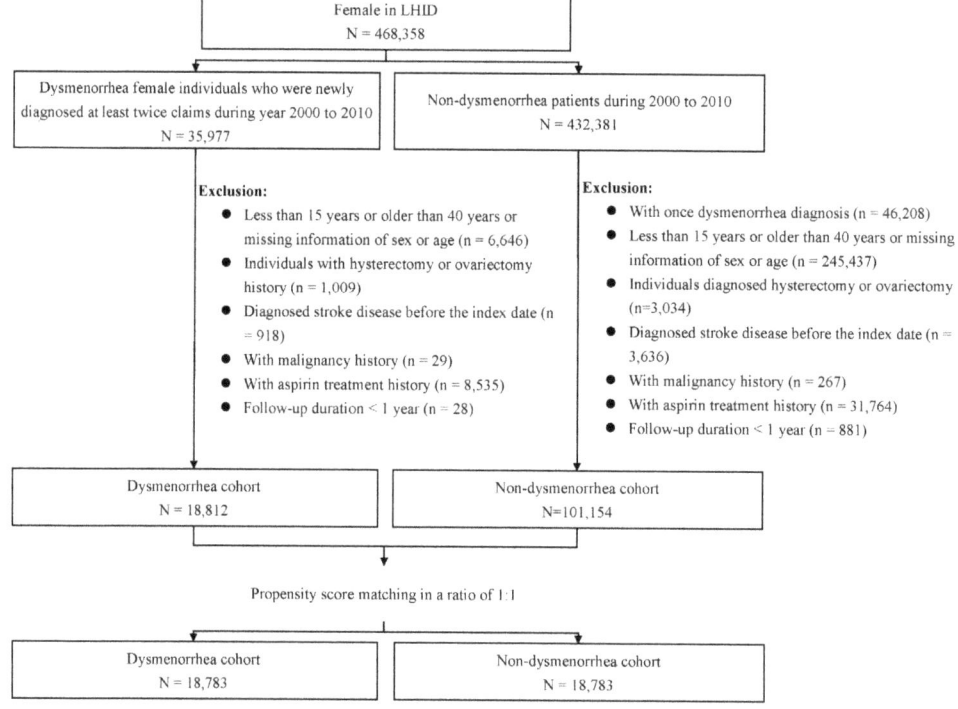

Figure 1. Flow chart for establishing study cohorts.

2.3. Outcome

Strokes that occurred shortly after inclusion in the study cohort may not have been associated with the risk factor. To adjust for the effect of immortal time bias, we began the follow-up one year after each individual's entry into the cohort. The follow-up person-years were counted up to the date the stroke (ICD-9-CM 430–438) was diagnosed, including hemorrhagic stroke (ICD-9-CM 430–432) and ischemic stroke (ICD-9-CM 433–438), or up to the date of withdrawal from the insurance program, or the end of 2013, whichever occurred first. The maximum follow-up period was 13 years.

2.4. Statistical Analysis

This study used SAS version 9.4 software (SAS Institute, Cary, NC, USA) to manage the data and perform the statistical analysis. A two-tailed *p*-value of less than 0.05 was considered to be statistically significant. Data analysis first compared the frequency distributions of age, comorbidities, and the use of non-steroidal anti-inflammatory drugs (NSAIDs) between the 2 cohorts. Women who had been prescribed NSAIDs for 10 days or longer were considered users. A chi-squared test was used to test the distribution of categorical variables between the two cohorts. Mean ages with standard deviations were compared between the two cohorts and tested using the *t*-test. We estimated and plotted the cumulative incidence proportions for overall stroke, ischemic stroke, and hemorrhagic stroke using Kaplan–Meier analysis. The log-rank test was used to examine the difference between the two cohorts. The incidence rate of stroke was calculated by dividing the number of stroke cases by the sum of follow-up person-years for each cohort. Cox proportional hazards regression analysis was used to estimate the PD cohort to the comparison cohort hazard ratio (HR) of stroke and the associated 95% confidence interval (CI). Age and comorbidity-associated HRs of stroke were assessed. We presented the Cox model estimated adjusted HR (aHR), which was estimated after controlling for matched pairs. We also presented results separately for ischemic stroke, hemorrhagic stroke, and the two stroke types combined together as the overall stroke. The likelihood ratio test was used to examine the interaction effects between the PD status and age, comorbidities, and NSAID.

3. Results

With similar sample sizes in the matched cohorts with and without dysmenorrhea (*n* = 18,783), distributions of age and comorbidities of both cohorts were similar (Table 1). With an average age of 25.5 years, 54% of the study population was aged 15–24 years. Thyroid disorders were the most prevalent among baseline comorbidities in both cohorts, whereas systemic lupus erythematosus and rheumatoid arthritis were the least common. Few women were taking NSAIDs for 10 days or longer.

Table 1. Distributions of age, comorbidities, and NSAID use compared between cohorts with and without primary dysmenorrhea.

Variable	Primary Dysmenorrhea				*p*-Value *
	No (N = 18,783)		Yes (N = 18,783)		
	n	%	*n*	%	
Age group (years)					0.99
15–19	524	26.8	5010	26.7	
20–24	5104	27.2	5134	27.3	
25–29	3635	19.4	3618	19.3	
30–40	5020	26.7	5021	26.7	
Mean (SD) [a]	25.5	(6.97)	25.5	(6.96)	0.93 [a]
Baseline comorbidities					
Diabetes mellitus	176	0.94	196	1.04	0.30
Hypertension	176	0.94	195	1.04	0.32
Hyperlipidemia	252	1.34	265	1.41	0.56
Obesity	90	0.48	116	0.62	0.07
Alcoholism	40	0.21	47	0.25	0.45
Arrhythmia	483	2.57	473	2.52	0.74

Table 1. Cont.

Variable	Primary Dysmenorrhea				p-Value *
	No (N = 18,783)		Yes (N = 18,783)		
	n	%	n	%	
Thyroid diseases	1162	6.19	1141	6.07	0.65
Migraine	640	3.41	640	3.41	1.00
Immune disorders	39	0.21	50	0.27	0.24
Systemic lupus erythematosus	12	0.06	22	0.12	0.09
Rheumatoid arthritis [b]	2	0.01	6	0.03	0.29 [b]
NSAID use					0.31
No	18,724	99.7	18,716	99.6	
Yes	59	0.3	67	0.4	

* chi-squared test. [a] t-test. [b] Fisher's exact test. NSAID, non-steroidal anti-inflammatory drug.

3.1. Overall Stroke

The Kaplan–Meier method estimated cumulative incidence of stroke after a maximum of the 13-year follow-up period was approximately 0.16% higher in the dysmenorrhea cohort than in the comparison cohort (0.88% vs. 0.72%) (log-rank test $p = 0.010$, Figure 2a), mainly contributed to by ischemic stroke (Figure 2b). The incidence rate of stroke was 1.51 times higher in women with dysmenorrhea than in the comparison cohort (6.05 vs. 4.01 per 10,000 person-years or 99 vs. 65 cases), with an aHR of 1.51 (95% CI 1.11–2.06) after adjustment for matched pairs (Table 2). The difference in incidence rates between cohorts was greater in the 25–40-year-old group (9.71 − 6.13 = 3.58 per 10,000 person-years) than in the 15–24-year-old group (3.02 − 2.25 = 0.77 per 10,000 person-years). The Cox method estimated PD cohort to comparison cohort HRs showed that none of the comorbidities had a significant role associated with stroke. There were no significant interaction effects between age and PD status and between each comorbidity status and PD status.

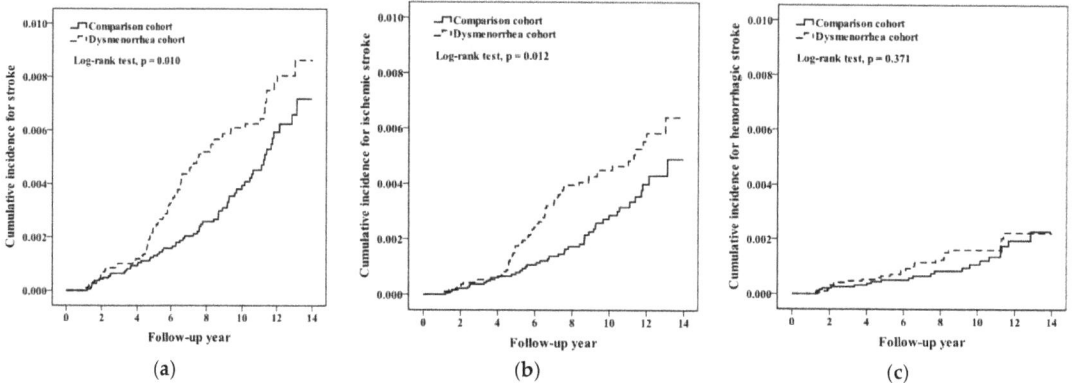

Figure 2. Kaplan–Meier method estimated cumulative incidence for (a) stroke, (b) ischemic stroke, and (c) hemorrhagic stroke in dysmenorrhea and comparison cohorts.

Table 2. Overall number of stroke events and incidence rates in primary dysmenorrhea and comparison cohorts by age, comorbidity, and NSAID use, and Cox model estimated primary dysmenorrhea cohort to comparison adjusted hazard ratio and 95% confidence interval.

Variables	Primary Dysmenorrhea							Hazard Ratio		p for Interaction
	No (N = 18,783)			Yes (N = 18,783)						
	Event, n	Person Years	Incidence Rate	Event, n	Person Years	Incidence Rate		Crude (95% CI)	Adjusted (95% CI)	
Total	65	162,247	4.01	99	163,625	6.05		1.52 (1.07–2.09) **	1.51 (1.11–2.06) **	
Age, year										0.63
15–24	20	88,807	2.25	27	89,478	3.02		1.36 (0.73–2.50)	1.34 (0.75–2.40)	
25–40	45	73,440	6.13	72	74,147	9.71		1.61 (1.08–2.32) *	1.58 (1.09–2.28) *	
Diabetes mellitus										0.96
No	62	160,771	3.86	99	161,922	6.11		1.60 (1.10–2.19) **	1.58 (1.16–2.17) **	
Yes	3	1476	20.33	0	1704	0.00		NA	NA	
Hypertension										0.06
No	57	160,814	3.54	94	161,963	5.80		1.65 (1.16–2.30) **	1.64 (1.18–2.27) **	
Yes	8	1433	55.84	5	1663	30.07		0.54 (0.13–1.66)	0.51 (0.16–1.61)	
Hyperlipidemia										0.34
No	64	160,444	3.99	94	161,565	5.82		1.45 (1.06–2.00) *	1.46 (1.06–2.00) *	
Yes	1	1803	5.55	5	2060	24.27		4.29 (0.29–44.2)	4.03 (0.47–34.7)	
Obesity										0.74
No	64	161,542	3.96	96	162,682	5.90		1.50 (1.02–2.11) *	1.49 (1.09–2.03) *	
Yes	1	705	14.18	3	943	31.81		2.31 (0.18–23.4)	2.01 (0.20–20.0)	
Alcoholism										0.97
No	63	161,981	3.89	99	163,267	6.06		1.58 (1.10–2.23) **	1.56 (1.14–2.13) **	
Yes	2	266	75.18	0	358	0.00		NA	NA	
Arrhythmia										0.96
No	62	158,292	3.92	99	159,573	6.20		1.60 (1.13–2.22) **	1.58 (1.16–2.17) **	
Yes	3	3955	7.59	0	4052	0.00		NA	NA	
Thyroid disease										0.51
No	62	152,380	4.07	92	153,816	5.98		1.48 (1.05–2.11) *	1.46 (1.06–2.01) *	
Yes	3	9867	3.04	7	9809	7.14		2.39 (0.44–9.86)	2.41 (0.64–9.04)	

Table 2. Cont.

Variables	Primary Dysmenorrhea						Hazard Ratio		p for Interaction
	No (N = 18,783)			Yes (N = 18,783)					
	Event, n	Person Years	Incidence Rate	Event, n	Person Years	Incidence Rate	Crude (95% CI)	Adjusted (95% CI)	
Migraine									0.94
No	62	157,425	3.94	94	158,629	5.93	1.53 (1.01–2.16) *	1.50 (1.09–2.07) *	
Yes	3	4822	6.22	5	4996	10.01	1.64 (0.26–7.11)	1.58 (0.37–6.71)	
Immune disease									1.00
No	65	161,878	4.02	99	163,037	6.07	1.53 (1.08–2.10) **	1.51 (1.11–2.06) **	
Yes	0	370	0.00	0	588	0.00	NA	NA	
NSAID use									1.00
No	65	161,735	4.02	99	163,041	6.07	1.53 (1.07–2.11) **	1.51 (1.11–2.06) **	
Yes	0	512	0.00	0	584	0.00	NA	NA	

Abbreviation: incidence rate, per 10,000 person-years; CI, confidence interval; NSAID, non-steroidal anti-inflammatory drug; NA, not applicable. Immune disease included immune disorders, systemic lupus erythematosus, and rheumatoid arthritis. p-values for hazard ratio: * < 0.05; ** < 0.01; p for interaction: p-value for interaction between dysmenorrhea status and stratified covariate.

3.2. Ischemic Stroke

The Kaplan–Meier analysis showed that the cumulative incidence of ischemic stroke during the follow-up period was approximately 0.15% higher in the dysmenorrhea cohort than in the comparison cohort (0.65% vs. 0.48%) (log-rank test $p = 0.012$, Figure 2b). Table 3 shows that the incidence rate of ischemic stroke in women with dysmenorrhea was 1.62 times higher than that in the comparison cohort (4.40 vs. 2.71 per 10,000 person-years or 72 vs. 44 cases), with an aHR of 1.61 (95% CI, 1.11–2.33) after adjustment for matching pairs. In addition, the difference in incidence rates between the two cohorts was greater in the 25–40-year-old group (7.82 − 4.08 = 3.74 per 10,000 person-years) than in the 15–24-year-old group (1.56 − 1.58 = −0.02 per 10,000 person-years). The ischemic stroke incidence rates in women with comorbidities were not all higher in women with PD. The Cox method estimated HRs also demonstrated that none of the comorbidities were significantly associated with stroke. There were no significant interaction effects between comorbidities and PD status.

3.3. Hemorrhagic Stroke

The Kaplan–Meier analysis shows that the cumulative incidence of hemorrhagic stroke during the follow-up was slightly higher in the dysmenorrhea cohort than in the comparison cohort by the follow-up year of 13 (log-rank test $p = 0.371$, Figure 2C).

Table 4 also shows that the hemorrhagic stroke incidence rate was slightly higher in women with dysmenorrhea than in the comparison cohort (1.65 vs. 1.29 per 10,000 person-years), with an aHR of 1.30 (95% CI, 0.74–2.29). The hemorrhagic stroke was not associated with the comorbidities.

Table 3. Number of ischemic stroke events and incidence rates in in primary dysmenorrhea and comparison cohorts by age, comorbidity, and NSAID use, and Cox model estimated primary dysmenorrhea cohort to comparison adjusted hazard ratios and 95% confidence intervals.

Variables	Primary Dysmenorrhea						Hazard Ratio		p for Interaction
	No (N = 18,783)			Yes (N = 18,783)					
	Event, n	Person Years	Incidence Rate	Event, n	Person Years	Incidence Rate	Crude (95%CI)	Adjusted (95%CI)	
Total	44	162,247	2.71	72	163,625	4.40	1.63 (1.07–2.35) *	1.61 (1.11–2.33) *	
Age, year									0.14
15–24	14	88,807	1.58	14	89,478	1.56	0.98 (0.44–211)	0.99 (0.47–2.07)	
25–40	30	73,440	4.08	58	74,147	7.82	1.91 (1.18–2.97) **	1.89 (1.22–2.92) **	
Diabetes mellitus									0.97
No	41	160,771	2.55	72	161,922	4.45	1.75 (1.12–2.60) **	1.73 (1.19–2.52) **	
Yes	3	1476	20.33	0	1704	0.00	NA	NA	
Hypertension									0.16
No	38	160,814	2.36	67	161,963	4.14	1.76 (1.12–2.63) **	1.73 (1.17–2.57) **	
Yes	6	1433	41.88	5	1663	30.07	0.72 (0.15–2.40)	0.68 (0.20–2.31)	
Hyperlipidemia									0.98
No	44	160,444	2.74	67	161,565	4.15	1.51 (1.01–2.32) *	1.50 (1.03–2.18) *	
Yes	0	1803	0.00	5	2060	24.27	NA	NA	
Obesity									0.78
No	43	161,542	2.66	69	162,682	4.24	1.58 (1.08–2.30) *	1.58 (1.08–2.30) *	
Yes	1	705	14.18	3	943	31.81	2.24 (0.18–22.3)	2.01 (0.20–20.0)	
Alcoholism									0.98
No	42	161,981	2.59	72	163,267	4.41	1.71 (1.04–2.51) **	1.68 (1.16–2.45) **	
Yes	2	266	75.18	0	358	0.00	NA	NA	
Arrhythmia									0.97
No	41	158,292	2.59	72	159,573	4.51	1.75 (1.10–2.61) **	1.73 (1.18–2.52) **	
Yes	3	3955	7.59	0	4052	0.00	NA	NA	
Thyroid disease									0.93
No	42	152,380	2.76	69	153,816	4.49	1.63 (1.07–2.40) *	1.61 (1.10–2.35) *	
Yes	2	9867	2.03	3	9809	3.06	1.52 (0.20–9.01)	1.50 (0.25–8.93)	
Migraine									0.63
No	42	157,425	2.67	67	158,629	4.22	1.61 (1.02–2.37) *	1.57 (1.07–2.30) *	
Yes	2	4822	4.15	5	4996	10.01	2.42 (0.40–13.2)	2.39 (0.46–12.4)	

Table 3. Cont.

Variables	Primary Dysmenorrhea								
	No (N = 18,783)			Yes (N = 18,783)			Hazard Ratio		p for Interaction
	Event, n	Person Years	Incidence Rate	Event, n	Person Years	Incidence Rate	Crude (95%CI)	Adjusted (95%CI)	
Immune disease									1.00
No	44	161,878	2.72	72	163,037	4.42	1.63 (1.04–2.41) *	1.61 (1.11–2.33) *	
Yes	0	270	0.00	0	588	0.00	NA	NA	
NSAID use									1.00
No	44	161,735	2.72	72	163,041	4.42	1.63 (1.01–2.44) *	1.61 (1.11–2.33) *	
Yes	0	512	0.00	0	584	0.00	NA	NA	

Abbreviation: incidence rate, per 10,000 person-years; CI, confidence interval; NSAID, non-steroidal anti-inflammatory drug; NA, not applicable. Immune disease included immune disorders, systemic lupus erythematosus, and rheumatoid arthritis. p-values for hazard ratio: * < 0.05; ** < 0.01; p for interaction: p-value for interaction between dysmenorrhea status and stratified covariate.

Table 4. Number of hemorrhagic stroke events and incidence rates in in primary dysmenorrhea and comparison cohorts by age, comorbidity, and NSAID use, and Cox model estimated primary dysmenorrhea cohort to comparison adjusted hazard ratios and 95% confidence intervals.

Variables	Primary Dysmenorrhea								
	No (n = 18,783)			Yes (n = 18,783)			Hazard Ratio		p for Interaction
	Event	Person Years	Incidence Rate	Event	Person Years	Incidence Rate	Crude (95%CI)	Adjusted (95%CI)	
Total	21	162,247	1.29	27	163,625	1.65	1.32 (0.70–2.37)	1.30 (0.74–2.29)	
Age, year									0.17
15–24	6	88,807	0.68	13	89,478	1.45	2.22 (0.70–5.98)	2.18 (0.83–5.76)	
25–40	15	73,440	2.04	14	74,147	1.89	0.96 (0.41–2.33)	094 (0.46–1.93)	
Diabetes mellitus									1.00
No	21	160,771	1.31	27	161,922	1.67	1.33 (0.68–2.40)	1.30 (0.74–2.29)	
Yes	0	1476	0.00	0	1704	0.00	NA	NA	

Table 4. Cont.

Variables	Primary Dysmenorrhea								Hazard Ratio		p for Interaction
	No (n = 18,783)				Yes (n = 18,783)						
	Event	Person Years	Incidence Rate		Event	Person Years	Incidence Rate		Crude (95%CI)	Adjusted (95%CI)	
Hypertension											0.98
No	19	160,814	1.18		27	161,963	1.67		1.36 (0.78–2.69)	1.34 (0.81–2.58)	
Yes	2	1433	13.96		0	1663	0.00		NA	NA	
Hyperlipidemia											0.98
No	20	160,444	1.25		27	161,565	1.67		1.40 (0.67–2.55)	1.37 (0.77–2.43)	
Yes	1	1803	5.55		0	2060	0.00		NA	NA	
Obesity											1.00
No	21	161,542	1.30		27	162,682	1.66		1.35 (0.66–2.70)	1.30 (0.74–2.29)	
Yes	0	705	0.00		0	943	0.00		NA	NA	
Alcoholism											1.00
No	21	161,981	1.30		27	163,267	1.65		1.34 (0.70–2.69)	1.30 (0.74–2.29)	
Yes	0	266	0.00		0	358	0.00		NA	NA	
Arrhythmia											1.00
No	21	158,292	1.33		27	159,573	1.69		1.32 (0.71–2.57)	1.30 (0.74–2.29)	
Yes	0	3955	0.00		0	4052	0.00		NA	NA	
Thyroid disease											0.28
No	20	152,380	1.31		23	153,816	1.50		1.19 (0.52–2.79)	1.15 (0.63–2.09)	
Yes	1	9867	1.01		4	9809	4.08		4.15 (0.34–44.9)	4.27 (0.54–34.1)	
Migraine											0.98
No	20	157,425	1.27		27	158,629	1.70		1.34 (0.66–2.72)	1.36 (0.77–2.42)	
Yes	1	4822	2.07		0	4996	0.00		NA	NA	
Immune disease											1.00
No	21	161,878	1.30		27	163,037	1.66		1.32 (0.64–2.57)	1.30 (0.74–2.29)	
Yes	0	370	0.00		0	588	0.00		NA	NA	
NSAID use											1.00
No	21	161,735	1.30		27	163,041	1.66		1.29 (0.66–2.59)	1.30 (0.74–2.29)	
Yes	0	512	0.00		0	584	0.00		NA	NA	

Abbreviation: incidence rate, per 10,000 person-years; CI, confidence interval; NSAID, non-steroidal anti-inflammatory drug; NA, not applicable. Immune disease included immune disorders, systemic lupus erythematosus, and rheumatoid arthritis. p for interaction: p-value for interaction between dysmenorrhea status and stratified covariate.

4. Discussion

In our study, the distributions of age and comorbidities at baseline were similar in the age- and propensity-score-matched PD cohort and the comparison cohort. We found that more than half of the PD patients were younger women aged 15–24 years, consistent with previous studies [6]. The incidence of stroke increased with age in our study population, which is consistent with the stroke in young women in the Netherlands [29]. We found age had an important role in the development of stroke. The difference of stroke incidence rates between the older and younger groups was near twofold greater in in the PD cohort than in the comparison group (6.69 vs. 3.88 per 10,000 person-years). The aHR of 1.34 for stroke was insignificant in women aged 15–24 years with PD. For women aged 25–40 years, the aHR of 1.58 for stroke was significant in women with PD, indicating that the older women with PD were at a higher stroke risk.

Some comorbidities increased stroke incidence and might be higher in the PD cohort than in the comparison cohort. However, the Cox method estimated PD cohort to comparison cohort HRs showed that none of these comorbidities were significant factors associated with stroke. The propensity score matching reduced the potential bias in stroke development associated with comorbidities.

In our study population, most prevalence rates of baseline comorbidities were less than 5.00%. Among the baseline comorbidities, the prevalence rates of thyroid disease were the highest in both cohorts, slightly lower in the PD cohort than in the comparisons (6.07% versus 6.19%). The disease was associated with a 2.3-fold higher incidence rate of stroke in the PD cohort than in the comparison cohort (7.14 vs. 3.04 per 10,000 person-years), but the numbers of associated stroke cases were few (seven versus three) and the aHR of depression for the PD cohort was not significant. Our data showed that the prevalence of hypertension in women with PD was slightly higher than that in the comparison cohort, which is consistent with the study conducted on women in Tianjin, China [30]. Women with hypertension had a higher incidence of stroke than women without hypertension in both cohorts. Interestingly, the hypertensive women in the PD cohort had a lower incidence of stroke than the comparison group. We suspect that the hypertensive women in the PD cohort could receive more medical attention to better control hypertension [31,32]. The benefit is insignificant, with an aHR of 0.51 (95% CI, 0.16–1.61) for stroke among hypertensive women in the PD cohort.

It is well known that ischemic stroke accounts for most strokes, nearly 70% to 80% of all strokes [29,33]. In the present study, ischemic stroke was also the main type of stroke in both cohorts. The PD cohort had a higher proportion of ischemic stroke than the comparison cohort (72.7% vs. 67.7%, or 72/99 vs. 44/66). The aHR of ischemic stroke was 1.61 (95% CI 1.11–2.33) for the PD cohort, mainly due to an elevated incidence rate in the older women. Women with PD may have increased thrombotic or embolic events that reduce blood flow to the brain [34,35]. Our data also showed that women with PD may be at higher risk for hemorrhagic stroke, but this was not significant, probably because of the small number of cases. It is unclear as to whether hypertension is associated with hemorrhagic events in women with PD. We suspect that the increased risk of stroke in women with PD is related to an imbalance of prostaglandins [36,37].

Women suffering from dysmenorrhea pain may experience a decreased quality of life [38,39]. NSAIDs may be prescribed to relieve the pain [21,28]. Studies have reported that long-term users of NSAIDs are at an increased risk of stroke, particularly hemorrhagic stroke [23,28,38,40,41]. A recent study examining the risk of stroke associated with NSAID uses for dysmenorrhea found that patients who took the medicine for 13 or more days per month were at an elevated risk of stroke. Those taking NSAIDs less than 13 days per month were at a lower risk of stroke with an aHR of 0.51 (95% CI 0.13–2.10) [42]. However, very few women had been prescribed NSAIDs for more than 10 days during the period with PD in this study. Therefore, the impact of this drug was not considered in our study.

There are some limitations in our study. First, PD is a common complaint among young women in our study. The finding is consistent with other Asian populations [9,15].

However, no study has investigated the stroke risk associated with PD for other Asian women. Second, it has been noted that the imbalance of hormones is not only related to dysmenorrhea but also affects the mechanism of estrogen in neuroprotection, reducing the risk of stroke [43]. Thus, women with dysmenorrhea have a higher risk of stroke than women in general. However, the insurance claims data provided no information on the laboratory data of hormones for evaluating the impact of estrogen. Third, a previous focus group study in Taiwan reported that young PD female patients used various self-care strategies, including diet, herbal remedies, and other complementary therapies [44]. Unfortunately, we could not evaluate the impact of these self-care treatments because they are not available in our database as well. Four, certain lifestyle information (smoking, alcohol consumption, exercise, and body mass index) is unavailable in the claims data and, therefore, could not be further adjusted in this study [45,46]. Finally, information on the severity of dysmenorrhea is not available to assess whether women with severe pain are at higher risk for stroke.

5. Conclusions

In this propensity score-matched follow-up study, we controlled for the effects of other comorbidities that might be associated with the risk of stroke. Our data showed that, with the exception of age, none of the comorbidities had a significant association with stroke risk for women with PD. Women with PD had an aHR of 1.51 for stroke compared to women without PD, mainly because of ischemic stroke. The age-specific data showed that the aHR of developing stroke in women with PD was significant for women aged between 25 and 40 years old, but not for those aged from 15 to 24, suggesting that healthcare providers may need to counsel women with dysmenorrhea with care strategies, particularly for older individuals.

Author Contributions: Concept or design of the study: C.-H.Y., C.Y.H. and F.-C.S. Data request: P.-S.Y., C.-H.M. and F.-C.S. Data analysis and interpretation: C.-H.M. and F.-C.S. Writing the draft: C.-H.Y. Revision of the article: F.-C.S. and C.Y.H. Funding: C.Y.H. Final approval for release: All authors. All authors have read and agreed to the published version of the manuscript.

Funding: This study is supported in part by Taiwan Ministry of Health and Welfare Clinical Trial Center (MOHW109-TDU-B-212-114004), MOST Clinical Trial Consortium for Stroke (MOST 108-2321-B-039-003-), Tseng-Lien Lin Foundation, Taichung, Taiwan.

Institutional Review Board Statement: This study was approved by the Research Ethics Committee of China Medical University and Hospital in Taiwan (CMUH104-REC2-115 (CR-4)).

Informed Consent Statement: Patient consent was waived because all identifications had been scrambled.

Data Availability Statement: All data are incorporated into the article.

Acknowledgments: We are grateful to Health and Welfare Data Center, China Medical University Hospital for providing administrative, technical, and funding support.

Conflicts of Interest: The authors declare no conflict of interest.

References

1. Karout, S.; Soubra, L.; Rahme, D.; Karout, L.; Khojah, H.M.J.; Itani, R. Prevalence, risk factors, and management practices of primary dysmenorrhea among young females. *BMC Women's Health* **2021**, *21*, 392. [CrossRef] [PubMed]
2. Hu, Z.; Tang, L.; Chen, L.; Kaminga, A.C.; Xu, H. Prevalence and Risk Factors Associated with Primary Dysmenorrhea among Chinese Female University Students: A Cross-sectional Study. *J. Pediatr. Adolesc. Gynecol.* **2020**, *33*, 15–22. [CrossRef] [PubMed]
3. Coco, A.S. Primary dysmenorrhea. *Am. Fam. Physician* **1999**, *60*, 489–496. [PubMed]
4. Latthe, P.; Latthe, M.; Say, L.; Gulmezoglu, M.; Khan, K.S. WHO systematic review of prevalence of chronic pelvic pain: A neglected reproductive health morbidity. *BMC Public Health* **2006**, *6*, 177. [CrossRef] [PubMed]
5. McKenna, K.A.; Fogleman, C.D. Dysmenorrhea. *Am. Fam. Physician* **2021**, *104*, 164–170. [PubMed]
6. Ju, H.; Jones, M.; Mishra, G. The prevalence and risk factors of dysmenorrhea. *Epidemiol. Rev.* **2014**, *36*, 104–113. [CrossRef]

7. Rogerio, A.; Lobo, M.; David, M.; Gershenson, M.D.; Gretchen, M.; Lentz, M.D. *Comprehensive Gynecology*, 7th ed.; Elsevier: Amsterdam, The Netherlands, 2017.
8. Abreu-Sánchez, A.; Parra-Fernández, M.L.; Onieva-Zafra, M.D.; Ramos-Pichardo, J.D.; Fernández-Martínez, E. Type of Dysmenorrhea, Menstrual Characteristics and Symptoms in Nursing Students in Southern Spain. *Healthcare* **2020**, *8*, 302. [CrossRef]
9. Ohde, S.; Tokuda, Y.; Takahashi, O.; Yanai, H.; Hinohara, S.; Fukui, T. Dysmenorrhea among Japanese women. *Int. J. Gynaecol. Obstet. Off. Organ Int. Fed. Gynaecol. Obstet.* **2008**, *100*, 13–17. [CrossRef]
10. Kazama, M.; Maruyama, K.; Nakamura, K. Prevalence of dysmenorrhea and its correlating lifestyle factors in Japanese female junior high school students. *Tohoku J. Exp. Med.* **2015**, *236*, 107–113. [CrossRef]
11. Chiu, M.H.; Wang, H.H.; Hsu, S.C.; Liu, I.P. Dysmenorrhoea and self-care behaviours among hospital nurses: A questionnaire survey. *J. Clin. Nurs.* **2013**, *22*, 3130–3140. [CrossRef]
12. Chiu, M.H.; Hsieh, H.F.; Yang, Y.H.; Chen, H.M.; Hsu, S.C.; Wang, H.H. Influencing factors of dysmenorrhoea among hospital nurses: A questionnaire survey in Taiwan. *BMJ Open* **2017**, *7*, e017615. [CrossRef] [PubMed]
13. Jung, H.S.; Lee, J. The effectiveness of an educational intervention on proper analgesic use for dysmenorrhea. *Eur. J. Obstet. Gynecol. Reprod. Biol.* **2013**, *170*, 480–486. [CrossRef] [PubMed]
14. Zhou, H.; Yang, Z. Prevalence of dysmenorrhea in female students in a Chinese university: A prospective study. *Health* **2010**, *2*, 311–314. [CrossRef]
15. Wong, L.P.; Khoo, E.M. Dysmenorrhea in a multiethnic population of adolescent Asian girls. *Int. J. Gynaecol. Obstet. Off. Organ Int. Fed. Gynaecol. Obstet.* **2010**, *108*, 139–142. [CrossRef] [PubMed]
16. Zhu, X.; Wong, F.; Bensoussan, A.; Lo, S.K.; Zhou, C.; Yu, J. Are there any cross-ethnic differences in menstrual profiles? A pilot comparative study on Australian and Chinese women with primary dysmenorrhea. *J. Obstet. Gynaecol. Res.* **2010**, *36*, 1093–1101. [CrossRef]
17. Samai, A.A.; Martin-Schild, S. Sex differences in predictors of ischemic stroke: Current perspectives. *Vasc. Health Risk Manag.* **2015**, *11*, 427–436. [CrossRef]
18. Redon, J.; Olsen, M.H.; Cooper, R.S.; Zurriaga, O.; Martinez-Beneito, M.A.; Laurent, S.; Cifkova, R.; Coca, A.; Mancia, G. Stroke mortality and trends from 1990 to 2006 in 39 countries from Europe and Central Asia: Implications for control of high blood pressure. *Eur. Heart J.* **2011**, *32*, 1424–1431. [CrossRef] [PubMed]
19. Tsao, C.W.; Aday, A.W.; Almarzooq, Z.I.; Alonso, A.; Beaton, A.Z.; Bittencourt, M.S.; Boehme, A.K.; Buxton, A.E.; Carson, A.P.; Commodore-Mensah, Y.; et al. Heart Disease and Stroke Statistics-2022 Update: A Report From the American Heart Association. *Circulation* **2022**, *145*, e153–e639. [CrossRef]
20. Rexrode, K.M.; Madsen, T.E.; Yu, A.Y.X.; Carcel, C.; Lichtman, J.H.; Miller, E.C. The Impact of Sex and Gender on Stroke. *Circ. Res.* **2022**, *130*, 512–528. [CrossRef]
21. Petrea, R.E.; Beiser, A.S.; Seshadri, S.; Kelly-Hayes, M.; Kase, C.S.; Wolf, P.A. Gender differences in stroke incidence and poststroke disability in the Framingham heart study. *Stroke* **2009**, *40*, 1032–1037. [CrossRef]
22. Reeves, M.J.; Bushnell, C.D.; Howard, G.; Gargano, J.W.; Duncan, P.W.; Lynch, G.; Khatiwoda, A.; Lisabeth, L. Sex differences in stroke: Epidemiology, clinical presentation, medical care, and outcomes. *Lancet Neurol.* **2008**, *7*, 915–926. [CrossRef]
23. Sohrabji, F.; Park, M.J.; Mahnke, A.H. Sex differences in stroke therapies. *J. Neurosci. Res.* **2017**, *95*, 681–691. [CrossRef] [PubMed]
24. Lin, M.H.; Yeh, C.H.; Mou, C.H.; Lin, Y.W.; Chen, P.C.; Chang, Y.Y.; Sung, F.C.; Wang, J.Y. Stroke risks in women with dysmenorrhea by age and stroke subtype. *PLoS ONE* **2019**, *14*, e0225221. [CrossRef] [PubMed]
25. Iacovides, S.; Avidon, I.; Baker, F.C. What we know about primary dysmenorrhea today: A critical review. *Hum. Reprod. Update* **2015**, *21*, 762–778. [CrossRef] [PubMed]
26. Yeh, C.-H.; Muo, C.-H.; Sung, F.-C.; Yen, P.-S. Risk of Ischemic Heart Disease Associated with Primary Dysmenorrhea: A Population-Based Retrospective Cohort Study. *J. Pers. Med.* **2022**, *12*, 1610. [CrossRef]
27. Kho, K.A.; Shields, J.K. Diagnosis and Management of Primary Dysmenorrhea. *JAMA* **2020**, *323*, 268–269. [CrossRef]
28. Ferries-Rowe, E.; Corey, E.; Archer, J.S. Primary Dysmenorrhea: Diagnosis and Therapy. *Obstet. Gynecol.* **2020**, *136*, 1047–1058. [CrossRef]
29. Ekker, M.S.; Verhoeven, J.I.; Vaartjes, I.; van Nieuwenhuizen, K.M.; Klijn, C.J.M.; de Leeuw, F.E. Stroke incidence in young adults according to age, subtype, sex, and time trends. *Neurology* **2019**, *92*, e2444–e2454. [CrossRef]
30. Xu, H.; Li, P.H.; Barrow, T.M.; Colicino, E.; Li, C.; Song, R.; Liu, H.; Tang, N.J.; Liu, S.; Guo, L.; et al. Obesity as an effect modifier of the association between menstrual abnormalities and hypertension in young adult women: Results from Project ELEFANT. *PLoS ONE* **2018**, *13*, e0207929. [CrossRef]
31. NCD Risk Factor Collaboration (NCD-RisC). Long-term and recent trends in hypertension awareness, treatment, and control in 12 high-income countries: An analysis of 123 nationally representative surveys. *Lancet* **2019**, *394*, 639–651. [CrossRef]
32. Pan, H.Y.; Lin, H.J.; Chen, W.J.; Wang, T.D. Prevalence, Treatment, Control and Monitoring of Hypertension: A Nationwide Community-Based Survey in Taiwan, 2017. *Acta Cardiol. Sin.* **2020**, *36*, 375–381. [CrossRef] [PubMed]
33. Vyas, M.V.; Silver, F.L.; Austin, P.C.; Yu, A.Y.X.; Pequeno, P.; Fang, J.; Laupacis, A.; Kapral, M.K. Stroke Incidence by Sex Across the Lifespan. *Stroke* **2021**, *52*, 447–451. [CrossRef] [PubMed]
34. Wardlaw, J.M.; Smith, C.; Dichgans, M. Small vessel disease: Mechanisms and clinical implications. *Lancet Neurol.* **2019**, *18*, 684–696. [CrossRef] [PubMed]

35. Tuttolomondo, A.; Daidone, M.; Pinto, A. Endothelial Dysfunction and Inflammation in Ischemic Stroke Pathogenesis. *Curr. Pharm. Des.* **2020**, *26*, 4209–4219. [CrossRef] [PubMed]
36. Ricciotti, E.; FitzGerald, G.A. Prostaglandins and inflammation. *Arterioscler. Thromb. Vasc. Biol.* **2011**, *31*, 986–1000. [CrossRef]
37. Wang, L.; Cheng, C.K.; Yi, M.; Lui, K.O.; Huang, Y. Targeting endothelial dysfunction and inflammation. *J. Mol. Cell. Cardiol.* **2022**, *168*, 58–67. [CrossRef]
38. Chen, C.X.; Draucker, C.B.; Carpenter, J.S. What women say about their dysmenorrhea: A qualitative thematic analysis. *BMC Women's Health* **2018**, *18*, 47. [CrossRef]
39. Patel, V.; Tanksale, V.; Sahasrabhojanee, M.; Gupte, S.; Nevrekar, P. The burden and determinants of dysmenorrhoea: A population-based survey of 2262 women in Goa, India. *BJOG Int. J. Obstet. Gynaecol.* **2006**, *113*, 453–463. [CrossRef]
40. Chang, C.H.; Shau, W.Y.; Kuo, C.W.; Chen, S.T.; Lai, M.S. Increased risk of stroke associated with nonsteroidal anti-inflammatory drugs: A nationwide case-crossover study. *Stroke* **2010**, *41*, 1884–1890. [CrossRef]
41. Park, K.; Bavry, A.A. Risk of stroke associated with nonsteroidal anti-inflammatory drugs. *Vasc. Health Risk Manag.* **2014**, *10*, 25–32. [CrossRef]
42. Lin, Y.W.; Wang, J.Y.; Lin, M.H. Stroke risk associated with NSAIDs uses in women with dysmenorrhea: A population-based cohort study. *PLoS ONE* **2021**, *16*, e0259047. [CrossRef] [PubMed]
43. Lisabeth, L.; Bushnell, C. Menopause and Stroke: An Epidemiologic Review. *Lancet Neurol.* **2012**, *11*, 82–91. [CrossRef] [PubMed]
44. Chen, C.H.; Lin, Y.H.; Heitkemper, M.M.; Wu, K.M. The self-care strategies of girls with primary dysmenorrhea: A focus group study in Taiwan. *Health Care Women Int.* **2006**, *27*, 418–427. [CrossRef] [PubMed]
45. Malek, A.M.; Cushman, M.; Lackland, D.T.; Howard, G.; McClure, L.A. Secondhand Smoke Exposure and Stroke: The Reasons for Geographic and Racial Differences in Stroke (REGARDS) Study. *Am. J. Prev. Med.* **2015**, *49*, e89–e97. [CrossRef]
46. Kadlecova, P.; Andel, R.; Mikulik, R.; Handing, E.P.; Pedersen, N.L. Alcohol consumption at midlife and risk of stroke during 43 years of follow-up: Cohort and twin analyses. *Stroke* **2015**, *46*, 627–633. [CrossRef]

Disclaimer/Publisher's Note: The statements, opinions and data contained in all publications are solely those of the individual author(s) and contributor(s) and not of MDPI and/or the editor(s). MDPI and/or the editor(s) disclaim responsibility for any injury to people or property resulting from any ideas, methods, instructions or products referred to in the content.

MDPI AG
Grosspeteranlage 5
4052 Basel
Switzerland
Tel.: +41 61 683 77 34

Journal of Clinical Medicine Editorial Office
E-mail: jcm@mdpi.com
www.mdpi.com/journal/jcm

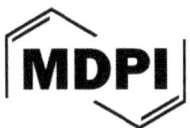

Disclaimer/Publisher's Note: The statements, opinions and data contained in all publications are solely those of the individual author(s) and contributor(s) and not of MDPI and/or the editor(s). MDPI and/or the editor(s) disclaim responsibility for any injury to people or property resulting from any ideas, methods, instructions or products referred to in the content.

www.ingramcontent.com/pod-product-compliance
Lightning Source LLC
LaVergne TN
LVHW070602100526
838202LV00012B/545